Personality and psychophysical health in relation to dance training A therapeutic intervention of dance movement therapy

By : Nagda, Leni

CONTENT

CHAPTER 1

INTRODUCTION

"There are short-cuts to Happiness and Dancing is one of them"

Vicki Baum

"The Job of feet is walking but their hobby is dancing"

Amit Kalantri

Dance has been a part of the human lives since ages. We perform dance for various purposes. We dance to celebrate, we dance to perform rituals, we dance to involve in recreational activities, we dance for fun, we dance for pursuing our hobby, we dance for artistic expression, we dance for getting physically fit, we dance to expression emotions, we dance to communicate and we dance to keep ourselves physical and mentally healthy. The sense of rhythm beats and dance is so effective that even babies respond to the tempo more than they do to the speech. It means human beings are born with the ability to move our body in response to the music

When we study the positive effects of dance on our health, some of the obvious and much discussed benefits include body flexibility, muscular strength, physical fitness, body balance and posture etc. Dance has also found to be effective in improving cognitions and memory, decreasing the risk of dementia. It also helps in overcoming depressive symptoms, dizziness, fatigue and procrastination. Dance has been found to be effective in creating new neural pathways due to which the information stored in the brain can be accessed with ease. It also results in more secretions of feel good neurotransmitters in our body. Dance is also an intensive activity for our brain through which various activities related to different senses are combined. The individual involves auditory, visual and tactile sensations along with the body balance, rhythm, coordination and movement.

Human beings have adopted a very fast and modern life style which has not only adversely affected their personality but has also resulted in occurrence of various psychosomatic disorders amongst them. According to an analysis by WHO, 60 % of the factors related with health and quality of life are related to the lifestyle.

Majority of people generally follow an unhealthy lifestyle leading to various illnesses and disabilities among them. People suffer from diseases and problems like hypertension, joint problems, metabolic diseases, anxiety, depression, cardio-vascular diseases, overweight etc. because of the adoption of an unhealthy life style. Atleast one out of every five people suffer from a mental illness globally. The problem has become so peculiar that it requires immediate attention and clinical concern.

Good health is essential to lead a longer and more active life. Good health has been be defined as a state of complete physical, mental and social well-being and not just absence of diseases, injury or pain. Alternatively, it may also be defined as being able to function in a manner it has been designed to function. It defines the functional efficiency or metabolic efficiency of an individual's mind, body and spirit and his ability to lead a socially and economically productive life. Physical health and mental health determine the efficiency of an individual hence, are the most discussed type of health. Physical health is critical for the overall well-being and is the most visible of the various dimensions of health, which include social, intellectual, emotional, spiritual and environmental health. Some of the most obvious and serious signs that we are unhealthy appear physically. Addressing this dimension is crucial for anyone attempting to sustain overall health and wellness.

PHYSICAL HEALTH

Physical health refers mainly to physical fitness. It is the overall physical condition of an individual at a particular time. Physical health may also be expressed as the soundness of the body, free from any disease or abnormality and the condition of optimal well-being. Physical health depends not only on genetic factors but also on economic, social and ecological factors. In other words, an individual's physical health depends to a large extent on his genes, but also on other factors like- where does he live, how clean or polluted is the air and water around him and how good is his social and medical system. A physically fit person would be able to walk or run miles without getting breathless and would be able to carry out his daily routine activities without any assistance. Generally the weight of a physically fit person is according to his height. He is neither underweight nor overweight. A taller person would have more weight compared to a short heighted person, but he would still be fit. If an individual is too heavy or too thin compared to his height, it may affect his health. This relation between hisweight and height is called the Body Mass Index (BMI).

Every individual wants to be healthy, but the environmental forces may attack his body or he may suffer from genetic malfunctions. To remain physically fit and maintain health,people need nutritious diet and physical activity (exercise). Physical activity helps people in reducing the risk of obesity, improving heart health and preventing many diseases. A healthy person is a quick healer. Human beings attain physical well- being generally by leading a healthy lifestyle which includes regular exercise, balanced and nutritious diet and adequate rest. Physical health also depends on the environment in which a person lives i. e exposure to sunlight or toxic substances also affects an individuals' physical health. Not drinking enough water may also cause headache and mood changes.Health is improved and maintained through the advancement and application of health science and through the efforts and intelligent lifestyle choices of the individual and society. According to the World Health Organization, the main determinants of health include the physical environment, social and economic environment, and an individual's characteristics and behaviors.

COMPONENTS OF PHYSICAL HEALTH

The vital components of physical health include muscular strength, flexibility of the body, cardiovascular endurance, body composition and muscular endurance among many other components.

Muscular Strength: refers to the power that enables people to lift and carry heavy objects. Without muscular strength, the body would remain weak and so an individual would not be able to perform his usual tasks efficiently. Muscular strength may be increased by doing regular workouts through different physical activities.

Flexibility of the body: Flexibility is yet another important component of physical health. Without flexibility, the muscles and joints of the body would become stiff which would restrict an individual's movement. A Flexible body can easily make various movements without pain or stiffness. Flexibility of the body may be checked by leaning forward and trying to touch the toes. People having a very flexible bodywould be able to touch their toes easily, while people who have less flexible bodywould not be able to touch their toes easily.

Cardiovascular Endurance: refers to the body's ability to take up physical activities like swimming, running, cycling, jogging whichenable the cardiovascular system (lungs, heart, blood vessels) to work for a longer period of time. Heart and the lungs fuel an individual's body with the oxygen required by muscles so that the body gets enough oxygen required for the work they are doing. The Cooper Run (running as far as possible in 12 minutes) is a test commonly used to assess cardiovascular endurance.Step Test (stepping onto a platform for 5 minutes) is also used by many trainers to measure anindividual's cardiovascular endurance.

Body Fat Composition: measures the amount of fat in a person's body. For instance, a person having a weight of 100-pounds and a 25% body fat composition would have a lean body mass of 75 pounds. According to body fat composition criteria, men having a body fat composition lower than 17 percent and Women with a body fat composition lower than 24 percent would be deemed fit.

Muscular Endurance: refers to the ability of muscles to perform contractions for extended periods of time. Instead of just lifting or carrying something for a few seconds, the muscles are used for minutes. To increase the strength of the muscles, people are initially given training with light weights which will train the muscle fibers needed for muscular endurance.

SOCIAL HEALTH

Social health enables people to behave and live collectively by effectively handling interpersonal relationships. It reflects ability of individuals to interact successfully in the global community. People need to develop their communication skills, their intimacy with others, and create a strong network of friends and family members to be social. Socially unhealthy people behave quite similar to people with mental and emotional problems. Socially healthy people discuss their sufferings with their friends and close people. Social health brings in societal changes.

ENVIRONMENT HEALTH

Environmental health controls the environmental factors that may negatively affect human life and people's health. It evaluates, corrects and controls the risk factors for human life. World Health Organization (WHO) has suggested three key factors that are a threat to health: poverty, excessive use of natural resources and the unsustainable economy. Environmental health not only helps a nation in saving energy and minimizing air pollution but also help to live in a cleaner and healthier environment.

MENTAL HEALTH

Mental health refers to an individual's emotional, psychological and social wellbeing. Good mental health is defined as the absence of anxiety, depression or any other disorder. It is a state of well-being where an individual is able to realize his or her own capabilities and is able to cope with the ordinary stresses of life to work productively and fruitfully. It may also be defined as a state of absence of mental illness. But actually mental health means much more than the absence of mental illness.Mental health is important at every stage of life, from childhood and adolescence through adulthood that is why a holistic approach to health – linking physical, mental, emotional and social health is essential for mental wellbeing. A mentally fit and stable person is able to balance various elements of his life viz. family, work and finances and feels more safe and secure.This approach also helps a great deal with managing and recovering from mental illness. Mentally healthy people experience a range of emotions such as joy, love, satisfaction. They easily cope with the challenges and changes of daily life and are aware how to seek help if they face difficulty coping with major conflicts, disturbances, traumas or transitions in different life cycles.

Physical health and mental health are strongly connected. Good physical health and mental health go hand in hand to improve an individual's overall quality of life. The Physical health status of an individual affects his mental health and wellbeing and mental illness of a person profoundly affects his physical health status. If people take care of their physical health, they automatically show an improvement in their mental wellbeing. On the contrary, poor physical health can lead to an increased risk of developing mental health problems. Similarly, poor mental health can negatively impact on physical health, leading to an increased risk of some conditions. People suffering from mental illness generally compromise their physical health. They are less focused towards their physical health care compared to those without mental illness. It has been a general observation that people involved with mental health services often overlook their physical health needs.

Key Physical Health Factors that promote Mental Wellbeing are-

- Balanced diet
- Adequate sleep
- Cutting down unhealthy habits such as drugs, smoking and alcohol.

Factors that have negative impact on mental wellbeing are-

- Stress
- Working too much
- Being too inactive.

Various ways in which poor mental health can have negative impact on physical health are-

- Mental illness such as anxiety and depression may cause excessive drug use disorders in an individual.
- People with a high level of distress have more probability of dying from cancer.
- Depression has a positive correlation with coronary heart disease (CHD).
- People suffering from mental illness are less concerned about their physical healthcare. They don't even get their routine checkups done (like blood pressure, weight and cholesterol) which might cause physical health problems in them at the later stage. They are also unable to give up smoking, reduce alcohol consumption and make positive changes in their diet.

Conditions recognized as mental illnesses are-

Mood disorders: also called affective disorders, such disorders involve persistent feelings of sadness or over happy. Feelings in such individuals fluctuate from extreme happiness to extreme sadness. The most common mood disorders are depression, bipolar disorder etc.

Psychotic disorders: refers to distorted thinking.The most common symptoms of such disorders are hallucinations, where a person sees some images or hears different sounds or voices that are not real. Delusionsrefers to some false beliefs that an individual accepts as real.

Eating disorders: is a situation which involves attitude, emotions and behavior related with food and weight. The most common eating disorders include anorexia nervosa, bulimia nervosa and binge eating disorder.

Personality disorders: People suffering from personality disorders have such inflexible personality traits in them which distresses them causing problems in their work, school, or social relationships. The thinking patterns and behavior of such people differssignificantly from the expectations of society and is so rigid that itintervenes with an individual's normal functioning. Example: antisocial personality disorder, obsessive-compulsive personality disorder, and paranoid personality disorder.

Impulse control and addiction disorders: People with such disorders are unable to resist their impulses or urges and do things that may be harmful to themselves or others. Kleptomania (stealing), Pyromania (starting fires) and compulsive gambling are examples of impulse control disorders. Often,such people have addiction of alcohol and drugs and they become so much addicted to their objects that they start ignoring their responsibilities and relationships.

Anxiety disorders: People suffering from such disorders respond to a situation or certain objects with fear. The physical signs of anxiety or panic such as a rapid heartbeat and sweating are clearly visible on their body. An anxiety disorder interferes with normal functioning of an individual. Anxiety disorders include generalized anxiety disorder, panic disorder, social anxiety disorder, and specific phobias.

PSYCHOSOMATIC DISORDERS

The word **psychosomatic** has been derived from two different words-**Psyche** which means mind and **soma** which means body. Psychosomatic disorder refers to the diseases concerned with the mind as well as body. At times the state of mental factors like stress and anxiety determines how severe would the physical disease be. Every physical disease has a mental aspect. How does an individual react to a disease and how would he cope up with it depends upon his mental state? For instance, rashes on the body may not bother some people very much while few others may start feeling depressed and ill due to such rashes.

Psychosomatic disorder is a condition in which psychological stress adversely affects the functioning of the body organs and the nervous system. A person scared of something may develop a feeling of anxiety. Psychosomatic disorders resulting from stress may include headache, hypertension, chest pain, irritability, pelvic pain, respiratory problems etc. Psychosomatic disorders or illness may originate or aggravate due to emotional stress and may emerge in the body as a physical pain or some other symptom. For instance, a person may suffer from back pain or high blood pressure due to stress in his daily life.

TYPES OF PSYCHOSOMATIC DISORDERS OR ILLNESSES

1. The first type of psychosomatic disorder an individual suffers from is mental illness as well as physical illness.

2. The second type of psychosomatic disorder an individual suffers from is that he faces a psychiatric issue due to some kind of physical illness. For instance, while taking the treatment of cancer, a patient may suffer from depression or anxiety.

PSYCHOPHYSICAL HEALTH

Psychophysical health refers to the physical health and mental health of an individual. Various elements of the psychological system are independent but function in an interlocking manner with physiological and other systems and keep changing gradually over a long period of time. Since every individual has a unique experience from life, therefore his reaction to the environment is also unique. His reaction to the environment depends to a large extent on his psychological traits and these traits enable him to make adjustments to the environment.For instance, identical twins born from the same fertilized egg, considerably vary in their behavior due to such unique aspects within them.

ANXIETY

Anxiety is a mental health disorder and a body's natural response to stress. A person may feel nervous while facing an interview, while giving a speech or before writing an exam. An individual having extreme feelings of anxiety, lasting longer than six months may suffer from an anxiety disorder.

ANXIETY DISORDERS

Anxiety disorders are types of mental illness that keeps a person away from carrying out a normal life. It is the most common form of emotional disorder and may affect anyone at any age. Such people usually face fear and worry but they start leading a normal life once they get their treatment. Anxiety disorders among people cause sleeplessness, heart palpitations, fear, panic, tense muscles etc. Ordinary anxiety is a normal feeling related to a situation that comes and goes but does not interfere with the life of an individual. On the contrary, in situation of anxiety disorder, a person may always suffer from the feeling of intense fear. Anxiety, if left untreated might get worse.

TYPES OF ANXIETY DISORDERS

Anxiety to a certain extent is normal, but excessive anxiety may lead to various kinds of anxiety disorders. Following are the types of anxiety disorders according to DSM IV TR.

Generalized Anxiety Disorder: This kind of anxiety disorder occurs due to excessive worry about everyday things. For instance, while going to work, a person may have worry that someone would throw a heavy object out of a window above, which would make him unconscious. No doubt, this event may occur but it is unlikely. Excessive fear for such events is very common among people with generalized anxiety disorder. Such people may also suffer from frequent heart palpitations or unwanted worrisome thoughts.

Obsessive Compulsive Disorder (OCD): This kind of anxiety disorder occur where an individual gets repeated, unwanted and irrational thoughts or fears in everyday life causing an individual to behave in a particular way. These constant thoughts or fears cause him to perform certain rituals or routines. The disturbing thoughts are termed as obsessions, and the rituals are called compulsions. For instance, a person going out of house for an hour is constantly worried that he may have left the stove on. Even after returning home and checking, the person is not convinced that the stove is off. A person with a fear of germs washes his hands constantly.

Panic disorder: It is a disorder where an individual suffers from recurring panic attacks. A person having panic disorder remains fearful all the time. Panic attacks cause a feeling of sudden terror in an individual. Though panic attacks subside in a short span of time, yet they result in people experiencing difficulty in breathing, feeling fatigued and unable to continue their day. A panic attack once or twice in a person's lifetime is normal but repeated attacks in a week or month are an indicator of panic disorder.

Post-Traumatic Stress Disorder (PTSD)**:** is a condition which develops when an individual experiences something unusual in his ordinary routine life or some traumatic andterrifying eventwhich shocks his world. For instance, sexual or physical assault, childhood abuse, the unexpected death of a loved one, rape etc. This disorder may be in the form of day dreams or nightmares and a person suffering from such a disorder may not be able to lead a normal life. Such a person would always suffer from anger and depression.

Social Anxiety Disorder: also known as social phobia**, it** is a situation where an individual suffers from extreme/ excessive fear of a specific situation, object or activity. It might be impossible for a person to leave his house due to the fear that he will be judged by others. People suffering from social phobia are generally not able to maintain their friendships, it's hard for them to hold down a job or go grocery shopping. Such people constantly worry about what others think of them and as a consequence they start avoiding social interactions.

All the above mentioned anxiety disorders reduce the ability of an individual to lead a normal and productive life. Such anxiety disorders would certainly require immediate treatment from trained professional to become manageable. Majority of people having an anxiety disorder get some relief after taking treatment and using these techniques in the long run may not disrupt their life.

There are changes in the classification of anxiety disorders in the DSM-V.

1. Anxiety Disorders - It includes separation anxiety disorder(excessive anxiety of separation from any beloved ones, home and even it is related to any pet also), selective mutism(complex childhood anxiety which is related to speak and communicate in some selected social settings), specific phobia(this is related to the fear of any specific object and place), social phobia(the fear of social gathering, to meet new people, talking to people), panic disorder(this is a anxiety of panic attack), agoraphobia(it involves avoidance of situations such as being alone outside of the home; traveling in a car, bus, or airplane; or being in a crowded area), and generalized anxiety disorder(it includes overly concerned about money, health, family, work, or other issues).

2. Obsessive - Compulsive Disorders- It includes obsessive-compulsive disorder (unreasonable thoughts and fears which are related to compulsive behaviors such as a fear of germs or the need to arrange objects in a specific manner), body dysmorphic disorder (this is a mental health disorder in which we can't stop thinking about one or more perceived defects or flaws in our appearance) , hoarding disorder(difficulty getting rid of possessions, leading to clutter that disrupts their ability to use their living or work spaces), trichotillomania(this is hair pulling disorder), and excoriation disorder(this is a skin picking disorder, in which the habit of skin picking cross its line).

3. Trauma and Stressor- It includes reactive attachment disorder(this is a condition in which a young child or an infant does not have emotional bond with his or her caretakers), disinhibited social engagement disorder(this is also a condition in which an infant and young child facing difficulty to develop meaningful connection with others, it may be because of their history of trauma, neglect etc.,), PTSD (It is Post-traumatic stress, stress after experiencing or witnessing any terrifying event) , acute stress disorder(it includes feeling of unpleasant, and dysfunctional reaction after an overwhelming traumatic event), and adjustment disorder(stress related conditions, it may create stress in routine work, at work place, at home and also with relationships).

DEPRESSION

Clinical depression refers to a mood disorder causing feelings of anger, sadness, loss or frustration in an individual. Such frequent mood swings may make an individual feel helpless and out of control. Depression may be caused due to several reasons. It might be due to prolonged illness, disappointment at home, work, or school, medical conditions, high blood pressure medications, alcohol or drug abuse, chronic stress, childhood events like abuse or neglect, social isolation (common in the elderly), nutritional deficiencies, sleeping problems and so on.

Depression may also cause psychosomatic disorder and may weaken an individual's immune system due to chronic stress. Such disorders require timely treatment just like other illnesses but unfortunately effective treatment does not get available to the patient on time and in an effective manner.

EFFECT OF PHYSICAL ACTIVITY ON PSYCHOPHYSICAL HEALTH

People need to be physically active to improve their overall health and fitness and prevent diseases. Physical activity means any movement of the body which involves using muscles and expands energy. From tending the garden to running a marathon, even gentle forms of exercise can significantly improve an individual's quality of life.Physical activity or exercise can improve health and reduce the risk of developing diseases like diabetes, cancer and cardiovascular disease. Regular physical activity is thus very effective in the primary and secondary prevention of several chronic diseases (e.g., cardiovascular disease, diabetes, cancer, hypertension, obesity, depression and osteoporosis) and premature death.

Various researches in the past have shown that a total of two-and-a-half-hour physical activity per week like brisk walking, playing basketball, swimming, running, cycling and dancing reduces the risk of many chronic diseases.

Aerobic activities also termed as endurance activities are a form of physical activities in which people move their large muscles in a rhythmic manner for a certain time with an aim to improve health or fitness. Aerobic activities reduce the risk of physical illnesses, improves the mood of a person and also improves his sleep. Physical activity also helps a person think more clearly as extra blood flows to the brain responsible for memory. Research shows that doing exercise influences the release and uptake of feel-good chemicals called endorphins in the brain. Even a short burst of 10 minutes brisk walking increases our mental alertness, energy and positive mood. Physical activity in form of an exercise results in –

- Muscle strength
- Bone Strength
- Prevention from diseases such as coronary heart disease, diabetes, cancer, osteoporosis, depression, High blood pressure, high blood cholesterol.
- Higher functional capacity.

Over time, regular physical activity makes the heart and cardiovascular system stronger.

WHAT IS DANCE?

Dance is a physical activity which involves a series of movementsmatching the speed and rhythm of music.It may also be defined asan activity in which people move rhythmically to music.It is a performing artwhich may be performed alone or in a group. Dance has been described in various ways and every human society has its own dances.Many people perform a dance to express their feelings and emotions or to feel better. Dance may also be used to express a story in front of the audience.In most of the societies, dance activity is performed with music. Most dances follow some style or pattern. For instance, couple dance is one such style, where a man and a woman dance together. Other form of dances needsa group of people to perform. While dancing a person puts all his emotions together,he is in his own world and nothing else then matters to him. He puts all his worries, frustrations, and stresses on hold. For a few moments, he is completely in the zone, where the music guideshim across the dance floor. Dancing makes people more disciplined,committed and develops their creative thinking skills.Through dance people learn not only about the music, rhythm and beat but also cooperative efforts required to produce a high quality work of art. Every person benefits from quality dance training. Dance is a great way to build invaluable social skills. It is an opportunity to teach people particularly children and adolescents the importance of movement and fitness in a variety of ways through a variety of disciplines. Dancers learn to take turns, to share attention, and to cooperate with others as they work within a group.Dancing is an activity through which dancers learn to coordinate muscles to move through proper positions.

Different styles of Dance:

- Classic dance
- Modern dance
- Jazz dance
- Ballet
- Samba
- Tango
- Rumba

- Hip hop
- Salsa
- Rock and Roll
- Folk Dance

Indian Classical Dances

- Kathak
- Kathakali
- Bharat Natyam
- Bhangara
- Kuchipudi

Dance is a universal activity, as it exists in most cultures across the world and can change its form to express different cultural meanings. Though dance is universal, it is affected by the numerous cultural influences, adaptations, and evolvement over time which changes the forms and varieties of dances.Expressive therapies like art therapy, play & drama therapy and music therapy allows individuals to express their thoughts and feelings without the need for a command on verbal communication. The therapeutic approaches to anxiety and depression through various Indian dance forms are a new entrant to dance literature. The Indian classical dances have been considered the dances of the mind and soul and are extremely traditional. This dance is a form of communication that brings out the innermost feelings and at the same time depicts the cultural aspects of a civilization. These dances reflect a spectacular and gorgeous aspect of the magnificent and continuous Indian dance tradition.

DANCE AND PSYCHOPHYSICAL HEALTH

Dance is another form of physical activity which may be used by therapists to treat psychosomatic disorders of human beings. Dance, as a physical activity, assists people of all ages to stay fit. Dance has a wide range of physical and mental benefits. Dance is considered a health promoting physical activity which assists in prevention and treatment of various physical and mental ailments. Dance as a healing art is as old as mankind, but it became an established profession in the early phase of twentieth century. Numerous studies in the past have revealed a considerable correlation between dance and psychological wellbeing.

Dance provides an active, non-competitive form of exercise that has potential positive effects on physical health as well as mental and emotional wellbeing. Dance offers several benefits to human beings including better conditions of the heart and lungs, weight management, increased muscular strength, stronger bones, improved mental functioning, greater self- confidence and self-esteem and improved social skills. Dance helps in strengthening the positive thinking of human beings. Apart from providing physical fitness, dance helps in weight control and stress reduction. Dance also increases the core strength of an individual's body which improves his body's balance, coordination, and posture and results in reduction of mechanical back pain.The Dance activity alone can in fact improve the mood and body satisfaction of an individual. Body movement, the most vital aspect of dance, simultaneously provides the means of assessment and the mode of intervention for dance/movement therapy.

Dancing, no doubt improves physical wellbeing of an individual, but at the same time it also improves his mental wellbeing. Dance has repeatedly shown positive impact on a person's mental health.

Dancing assists an individual in improving his mood swings and reduce his stress and anxiety. Dance releases abundance of mood-improving chemicals in the body of a dancer. These chemicals improve one's mental state to such an extent that even a single session is able to reduce depression. Several studies prove that despite problems such as stress, depression and anxiety, dance can result in high positive experience for the participants.The participants who took the dance classes had improved mental health and a boost in mood compared to those who did not take the dance classes. The positive effects of dance activity lasted up to eight months after the classes ended. Hip hop dance, for instance, lowers the level of stress in addition to boosting energy and mood.

DANCE AS A SOURCE OF DEPRESSION AND ANXIETY REDUCTION

Dance is one of those beneficial activities which is frequently included in recommendations to address anxiety and depression. With the help of Dance one can decrease the level of Anxiety, Stress and depression. A study conducted by the

University of Oxford reveals that patients suffering from anxiety and depression showeda measurable level of reduction in their depression when they were involved in recreational dance sessions.Even dances which involve physical contact between people through touch, reduce the levels of stress and anxiety, leading to an individual's overall mental wellbeing.

PERSONALITY

Personality refers to the characteristics or qualities of an individual that differentiate him from other individuals and make him recognizable as a distinct character. Personality may be defined as the sets of behaviors and emotional patterns that evolve from biological and environmental factors. Personality encompasses all the traits and characteristics that distinguish an individual from others.The assessment of the qualities or characteristics of an individual is being done using various personality traits, which constitute the most basic unit of individual's personality. Trait-based personality theories define personality as the traits that predict an individual's behavior. On the contrary, other behavior-based approaches define personality through learning and habits. The personality traits are determined by the action, attitude and behavior of an individual. The personality traits guide and direct behavior of individual and enable them behave in aparticular manner. Traits are found within the individual and can be verified empirically. It has generally been observed that people belonging to the same country or a community within society behave in a similar manner in a number of situations. This is due to the fact that cultural factors have a very significant role in the development of personality. They usually hold the same viewpoints and behave in like manner as others.

Personality traits may be positive or negative. For instance, patience and loyalty are positive personality traits. Being honest and responsible are again positive traits of a personality. Negative personality traits could be like being disloyal, being quick to anger, being rigid and selfish etc. Personality of an individual has psychological aspects as well as physical aspects. The interacting factors at the physiological level include the endocrine system and the various glands in the system. The interacting factors at the psychological level includes emotions, traits, character, intellect, temperament etc. These psychological aspects interact with the physiological aspects and contribute to the personality behavior and development.

The researchers at the Personality Project definepersonality as the coherent pattern of cognition, affect and desires (goals) because all these lead to behavior. Personality may be defined in different ways, depending on whether the personality of an individual or a group of people in general is being described. If the personality description focuses on people in general, then the personality may be defined in terms of individual differences — that is, the wide range of different styles of thinking, feeling and acting. Just like human beings may differ a great deal in terms of their physical traits (height, weight, hair, and so on), similarly they may also differ in their mental and behavioral traits. For instance, some people are noticeably talkative and outspoken while others are noticeably reserved and quiet. Such variations and differences may be seen everywhere throughout the human population. If we focus on the personality of an individual, we can define it as a set of enduring dispositions or long-term tendencies to think, feel and act in particular ways.

Study of the psychological aspect of a personality, termed as personality psychology, attempts to explain the tendencies that cause differences in behavior among the individuals. Various approaches viz. cognitive, humanistic, biological, learning and trait-based theories and psychodynamic have been used to study personality.

PERSONALITY TRAITS: BIG FIVE PERSONALITY THEORY

The personality of an individual can be measured using several ways, but psychologists prefer to measure a person's personality on the basis of personality traits. According to psychologists, the most popular personality framework is the Big Five, also called the five-factor model of personality. Five vital traits that describe a personality are introversion/extroversion, openness, conscientiousness, extraversion, agreeableness and neuroticism. Due to the popularity of this theory of personality, it is applicable to people in many countries and cultures around the world, it provides a reliable assessment scale for measuring personality.These five factors do not provide completely exhaustive explanations of personality, but they are known as the Big Five because they encompass a large portion of personality-related terms. The five factors are not necessarily traits in and of themselves, but factors in which many related traits and characteristics fit.

For example, the factor agreeableness encompasses terms like generosity, amiability, and warmth on the positive side and aggressiveness and temper on the negative side. All of these traits and characteristics (and many more) make up the broader factor of agreeableness.

Openness to experience: is one of the five personality traits given in the Big Five personality theory which indicates how open-minded an individual is. It is also termed as intellect or imagination sometimes.It has been observed that individuals who reveal high level of opennessin the personality testgenerally enjoy trying new things,thinking outside the box and adventurous life. They are not only open-minded but also imaginative and curious. They appreciate art, imagination and new things. They believe in the fact that Variety is the spice of life.

Individuals low in openness in the personality test are just the opposite. They generally don't prefer trying new things rather prefer to stick to their habits and avoid new experiences. Such kind of people are usually close-minded and enjoy having a routine.

Changing an individual's personality is usually considered a difficult process, but openness is a personality trait that is subject to change in adulthood.

Common traits related to openness to experience include:

- Cleverness
- Curiosity
- Daring
- Ability to be vulnerable
- Creativity
- Intellect
- Preference for variety

Conscientiousness: another crucial personality trait given by theBig Five personality theory. Generally an individual scoring high in conscientiousnesspersonality testis a self-disciplined personality, organized and has a strong sense of duty. These individuals don't act spontaneously, rather do everything in a planned manner. They're dependable and achievement-focused. Systematic planning by such individuals makes them highly successful in their chosen occupation. Such individuals are highly responsible and reliable. People low in conscientiousness are more spontaneous. They may tend toward carelessness. Conscientiousness is a trait which has been linked to achievement in school and on the job.

Traits within the conscientiousness factor include:

- Hard work
- Reliable
- Ambitious
- Resourcefulness
- Perseverance
- Energetic

Extraversion: Extraversion and introversionare the most recognizable personality trait of the Big Five. Extraversion is a personality trait that indicates how outgoing and social a person is. The more extravert an individual is, the more social he is. Extraverted behaviors include being talkative, adventurous and assertive. Extraverts are chatty, sociable and draw energy from crowds. They tend to be assertive and cheerful in their social interactions. Extraverts tend to be happier than introverts. This concept has been explained by two theories- instrumental theories and temperamental theories. According to the instrumental theory, extraverts make such choices which puts them in more positive situations and they also react more strongly compared to introverts in positive situations. On the contrary, the temperamental theory believes that extraverts possess certain qualities which enable them experience a higher degree of positive affect. Individuals scoring high in extraversion in the personality test are those who enjoy the company of people, participate frequently in social gatherings and are full of energy. They enjoy engaging with the external world.

A person low in **extraversion** is less outgoing and more comfortable working on his own. He enjoys his own company and doesn't mingle with people frequently. Introverts, need plenty of time alone, because their brains process social interaction differently. Introverts can be perfectly charming at parties, but otherwise they prefer solo or small-group activities.Introversion is often confused with shyness, but both the terms have a different meaning. Shyness implies a fear of social interactions or an inability to function socially. In general, extroverts draw energy from or recharge by interacting with others, while introverts get tired from interacting with others and replenish their energy with solitude.

The traits associated with extroversion are:

- Talkative
- Sociable
- Fun-loving
- Friendly
- Assertive
- Confident
- Affectionate

Agreeableness is a personality trait in individuals that makes him a kind, sympathetic and cooperative person. **Agreeableness** measures the extent of a person's warmth and kindness. The more agreeable someone is, the more likely they are to be trusting, helpful and compassionate. This personality trait differentiates an individual in terms of cooperation and social harmony. People scoring high in agreeableness in the personality test are empathetic, are judged to be better dancers while individuals scoring low reflect selfish behavior of individuals and a lack of empathy. Those who score very low on agreeableness show signs of competing with others rather than cooperating.

Disagreeable people are cold and suspicious of others, and they're less likely to cooperate.

The following traits are associated with agreeableness:

- Trust
- Kind
- Humbleness
- Polite
- Loyal
- Patience

- Modest
- Helpful
- Cheerful

Neuroticism: People high in neuroticism worry frequently and easily slip into anxiety and depression. Even if all goes well, neurotic people tend to worry about everything. A study by various researchers in 2012 revealed that when the salaries of neurotic people increased, the additional income earned by them made them less happy. In contrast, people who are low in neuroticism tend to be emotionally stable and even-keeled. Neuroticism is linked with plenty of bad health outcomes. Neurotic people die younger than the emotionally stable, because they start consuming tobacco and alcohol to ease their nerves.

Traits commonly associated with neuroticism:

- Nervous
- Jealous
- Pessimist
- Insecure
- Oversensitive
- Lack of confidence
- Instable
- Anxiety

PSYCHOTHERAPY

Psychotherapy refers to the use of psychological methods to assist a person change his behavior and overcome problems in an effective way. Psychotherapy aims to improve an individual's quality of life by improving his physical and mental health. It aims to mitigate troublesome behaviors, beliefs, thoughts, or emotions of individuals and improve their relations with their family, relatives, friends and colleagues.

Some psychotherapies such as sand play have been specifically designed for children and adolescents to make them stress, depression and anxiety free individuals.

Various psychotherapy techniques have evolved over the years aiming to mitigate mental disorders due to stress, anxiety and depression. These therapies are generally utilized by the psychotherapists who may be mental health professionals such as psychiatrists, psychologists, mental health nurses family therapists, or professional counselors.

DANCE MOVEMENT THERAPY (DMT)

The dance movement therapy is a therapy which has recently emerged in the field of psychotherapy. Dance movement therapy falls into the category of expressive therapy. Therapists use expressive therapies with a belief that each individual has a different expressive styles, such as visual, and tactile (Levy, 2005). Generally, the dance/movement therapists, use these dance movements to help the clients heal and express their feelings. Many people who suffer from some kind of mental illness are usually unable to express their feelings. However with the help of dance, individuals are comfortably able to express themselves. The dance therapy works on the concept of using the body as a tool to express emotions and feelings to others.

The present research study aims to explore how the dance movements and dance training therapy may be utilized by therapists to reduce the clinical symptoms of mental illness, and improve overall health and wellbeing. The Dance/movement therapy (DMT), has recently gained popularity and recognition as an effective instrument in decreasing the mental and physical illness. Dance movement therapy has been acknowledged as a more comprehensive approach to the management of mental health symptoms. The therapy is based on the idea that body and mind are co-relational i.e., very closely related to each other.

Dance movement therapy is a movement based psychotherapeutic approach which uses body movements to inculcate emotional, social, cognitive and physical completion in the individuals to enhance health. While analyzing the effectiveness of DMT, various authors haveexplained that dance not only enhances the quality of life of individuals but also decreases clinical symptoms of depression and anxiety. Thus, this research study endeavors to evaluate the effectiveness of the therapeutic use of dance as a psychological treatment for the psychological problems. Most DMT professionals work in psychiatric hospitals, rehabilitation centers, and schools. Some DMT professionals also carry on their private practice through their private clinics.

Though there has been a lot of qualitative research in DMT, yet in recent years, evidence based quantitative research is becoming popular.

Dance therapy is a therapy that uses body movements to assist individuals achieve physical, emotional, cognitive and social integration. The therapy is beneficial for stronger physical health as well as mental health. Dance therapy is used by the therapists for stress reduction, disease prevention, and mood management of their clients. The physical component of DMT results in increased muscular strength, decreased muscular tension, coordination and mobility. The therapy may be used with all populations and with individuals, couples, families, or groups. In general, dance therapy enhances the self-awareness and self-esteem of people which enables them express their feelings.

The Dance Movement Therapy works on the following assumptions:

1. Body, mind and spirit are interconnected and a change in one impacts the other.
2. Movement is a language for communication: Therapists believe that nonverbal language i.e communication through gestures and movements is as important as verbal language as people are able to express themselves in a better way through gestures and movements.
3. Movement also acts as an assessment tool: By observing the movements of an individual, therapists are able to assess their mental state. Dance movement therapists also use body movements in their psychotherapeutic work.
4. Movements help people concentrate better, sleep better, have more energy and become resilient when they are facing any emotional or mental issue. Regular movements is an investment for their body, mind and soul. DMT is thus the psychotherapeutic use of various movements and dance to control and affect the emotional, physical and mental functions of an individual's body.
5. Movements can be symbolic and are able to express various aspects of the personality.
6. Movement improvisation and experimentation makes individuals more expressive and develop them into a new personality.

Dance movement therapy helps –

- To restore body's optimal mechanism.
- cleanse the toxins accumulated in the body due to lifestyle choices.
- repairs the cells, tissues and all affected parts of the body and rejuvenates the system.
- the individual in focusing on what he/she can do, rather than he/she cannot.
- brings out individual's own will and inner potential to live well.
- heightens sense of awareness of his/her body and mind to restore his/her emotional and physiological wellbeing.

DANCE MOVEMENT THERAPY FOR ANXIETY DISORDERS

Various researches and studies have demonstrated that dance therapy can be very effective in the treatment of mental health issues like depression, disordered eating and anxiety.Anxiety disorder is a very serious mental ill health worldwide. Though interventions such as Dance Movement Therapy(DMT) offer several treatment options for anxiety disorders , the clinical guidelines do not accept these interventions due to lack of sufficient research.There are ample empirical evidences through various rigorous research studies that depression and anxiety not only cause health risks to individuals, but also involve several psychosocial risks. People suffering from anxiety and depression have a greater risk of social and psychological problems, such as discrimination and poor self-esteem, which can continue in their lives for a very long period. Such kind of people are more likely to suffer from sadness, loneliness and nervousness. In addition, these people are often the target of peer-victimization i.e teasing and bullying and social discrimination. The psychological stress of social discrimination causes low self-esteem which, in turn, may hinder their academic and social functioning.

The present study conducted a systematic study to explore the effectiveness of DMT with people with anxiety disorders.According to some psychologists and therapists, Dance has had a very effective response on healing the anxiety disorders. For this reason, many therapists who treat anxiety find dance as an effective and potential treatment for anxiety. Dancing was found to help anxiety and depression victims embrace their bodies and feel safe in their own bodies again (Leseho & Maxwell, 2010).

Dance helps an individual not only explore his creativity but also be in the state of peaceful mind. It has been observed by therapists that people suffering from anxiety disorders often face difficulties in intra-personal and interpersonal relating. Therapists also observed that dance therapy created a positive change in the patients with anxiety disorders.DMT is actually considered effective in cases when people need to overcome anxiety disorders. DMT is used by therapists to address relational issues and emotional issues of individuals and help them rehabilitate. Therapists use body of individuals as an instrument to stop the feelings of anxiety disorders, to re-energize their body powers and to enhance their mind working. Dance Movement Therapy, as a psychotherapy has proved to be very effective in the modern world in reducing the anxiety disorders as well as mental illness. It also enables an individual lead a normal life and achieve his dreams and wishes. The DMT sessions include process of observation, assessment, interventions, verbal processing etc. Sessions may be highly structured and may be conducted individually or in groups.

DANCE MOVEMENT THERAPY IN PERSONALITY DEVELOPMENT

DMT is not only effective in treating various mental diseases but it has a very positive impact on a person's physical health and personality development. Dance is an embodied activity and when it is applied therapeutically, it leads to several health benefits. Not only this, dance is a very crucial activity to bring in personality transformation in an individual. According to various researches in the past, Dance as a physical activity created not only a feeling of joy among the individuals but also improved their self-expression.Dance movement therapy (DMT) is a process which helps the patients recognize and express their feelings. The Body movements of a person reflect his inner psychic life and his relationships with the outside world. Dance therapy works on the assumption that body and mind are interrelated. Dance therapists are of the opinion that mental and emotional problems present in the body of an individual restrict his movement patterns. A dance therapist may not be well versed with dance techniques, yet he treats his patients by observing how a person feels his body and movement.

Dance therapists use this versatile form of therapy and work with people to help them improve their body image and self-esteem. The creative expression of Dance therapy is widely used to improve communication skills and dynamic relationships. Dance therapy works on the idea that motion and emotion are interconnected. The therapy solves the following issues of an individual-

Physical Issues:

- Hypertension
- Arthritis
- Cardiovascular disease
- Chronic pain

Mental Health Issues:

- Anxiety
- Posttraumatic stress
- Poor self-esteem
- Depression
- Disordered eating

Cognitive Issues:

- Dementia
- Communication issues

Social Issues:

- Family conflict
- Domestic violence trauma
- Aggression

Stages of Dance Movement Therapy:

Dance movement therapy is a type of creative process which can be bifurcated into four stages and each of these stages should be composed of smaller set of goals. The goals thus made should be accompanied with the broad purpose of the therapy and these goals should be varies and changes from person to person depending on the need of the individual. The stages thus divided should be progressive in nature. However, while completing the whole therapy the patient may be visited many times depending on the need. Here, we are discussing these four stages in detail so as to get idea about theses stages:

- Preparation: In this stage the central theme is to establish safety with the help of doing warm-up this is the reason this stage is also known as warm-up stage.
- Incubation: This stage is followed by warm-up stage and in this mainly relaxation is focused as in this the person is allowed to let's go off with his consciousness control due to this his symptoms become symbolic.
- Illumination: this is the third stage in which the outcomes become evident which can be negative or positive.
- Evaluation: This is the last stage and in this the benefits of the whole process is discussed with the person who is undergoing in this process and after this the therapy comes to an end.

Dance Therapy Techniques and Benefits:

There are various types of dance and movements' activities and techniques are available which can be utilised by dance therapist while addressing client needs. Some of the examples of these techniques are discussed here

- ***Mirroring:*** For showing empathy and validating feeling of person matching and echoing movements is done and for the above purpose therapist may mirror a client's movements or he can ask to clients to have mirror for one another so as to enable them to see reflection of themselves.
- ***Movement metaphors:*** For physically and expressing demonstrating therapeutic challenge or achievement movement metaphor or movement can help in the same for example: the therapist may provide a white flag to the person for celebrating emotional surrender.
- ***Jumping rhythms:*** The therapist may include jumping into dance for the patients who are experiencing depression as it is seen in the researches that the vertical movements are helpful in people suffering from depression.

Some other techniques of dance-movement therapy have been discussed in Chapter-3 along with the discussion on intervention model of DMT proposed by the researcher.

Some of the important skills can be acquired during the dance movement dance therapy process. Here, we have discussed short list of these skills:

- It helps in learning in how to develop and trust your abilities to be present empathetically
- In making able oneself in responding authentically and truthfully.
- In learning that how to translate the non-verbal movements into insights which is utilised in recovery

Feelings and life experiences are present inside the body which can get trapped inside body. The body can be used as a key in unlocking profound level of healing. DMT is not a dance class but a therapeutic exposure and when it is provided in conjunction with other therapies helps in accessing more genuine and long-lasting change.

Factors which may be involved in some of the DMT sessions are:

1. For observation, assessment, communication and interaction and also for treatment dance and movement therapy are used for entire therapeutic processes.
2. The sessions are likely to be start with warm-up which is followed by cool-down.
3. Usually, therapist will motivate one to explore the various forms of movement so as to improve the growth.
4. Sometimes music is also utilised to accompany dance.
5. To make one understand some of his/her movements therapist may mirror some of the movements so one can experience and communicate their understanding of it as the therapeutic understanding is central theme in DMT.
6. For building a better awareness in terms of his/her body the therapist can help in this by utilising movement or dance. in this process they can instruct to make a particular gesture or to make changes in the gesture or they can observe mindfully.

7. One can develop a sequence of movements or dance which is based on the choices of him/her depending on the inner experience as it is seen that this therapy is helpful in working with different emotions.

8. While at the finishing of the sessions, the therapist can ask one about experience related to the sessions or can assist him/her in connecting with nonverbal experience with words.

Characteristics of Dance Movement Therapist:

1. ***Courage:*** It is one of the most important characteristics that a dance therapist should have in them as it takes a lot of courage to dance shamelessly around your clients. Although some good music and knowledge helps in facilitating therapeutic changes but the major factor which is to be more focused is the relationship between the client and therapist and that's the most terrific thing and it takes lot of courage to get up and ask – "What would everyone liketo do in dance movement therapy?". And then would see that where the groups would like to go.

2. ***Body awareness:*** we can say that it is the precursor that a dance therapist should possess is that they should have body awareness and as it is seen that the dancers are aware about their bodies so we can say that dance therapist should be former dancer as they usually have body awareness. The dance therapists are one step further in having body awareness because the dance therapist should understand what actually body wants to tell? The dance therapist should have a vast knowledge of body awareness as it is one of major factors which helps in making therapy beneficial and successfully.

3. ***Mindfulness:*** The therapist should have present mind due to the multiple reasons as it helps in intervention choices, to understand the feeling of the client and assist in body awareness and help in co-ordinating between mind and body also it promotes self-care.

4. ***Improvisational skill:*** These skills play a very significant role in Dance/ Movement therapy and the therapist should have these skills in order to improve and making therapy more beneficial. For example: there is already a lot of discussion about mirroring in dance movement therapy and by following the same sessions in the repeating mode may leads to develop boringness and cannot give a desirables result. For avoiding this complication, one should think about different ways to improve the therapy and this is the place where improvisational skills works and the therapist can impress client and produce desirable results.

5. ***The understanding that you won't be ever same:*** The therapist should understand that after learning dance/movement therapy they will change a lot and they can build their introspective nature of learning and this leads for them to become a dance/movement therapist.

6. ***The ability to get out of your own way:*** The therapist should know the ways to get out of the problems in their own way as the therapy is a dynamic process one need not to be worry about doing wrong things instead, they should possess the skill to get out of the problems as all the things happens in therapies are informative and valid and are very important experience. All therapists need to know how to get out of the problems they faced during therapy.

7. ***Flexibility:*** As we know the dance/movement therapy jobs are intense because it requires continuous body/mind processing and being flexible is one of the best ways to combat stress. It is well known that the DMT varies from person to person and a single therapy does not fit for all so the dance therapist needs to be flexible which helps them to serve their client in best way.

8. ***Kindness:*** In order to do this work or nay mental health profession one should be kind. The therapist should be kind which transcends their action and interaction to the external world and also, they should be kind in their DMT community as it is very small community.

Conclusion

Both Dance and Dance Movement therapy differ on many grounds. Dance is done for leisure or pleasure even if it may be effective in providing certain health benefits. Dance Movement therapy on the other hand is more about providing the clients the opportunity to express their emotions. DMT is a type of psychotherapy which has definite goals and intervention and treatment plan. In dance, there can be an instructor, but in DMT, there is always a facilitator. Both dance and dance movement therapy may help in developing self confidence, self concept, self esteem and other mental health parameters but the process through which both reach to the goals are significantly different. Dance focuses on the skills, techniques, and steps and is more about the end product that is the learnt dance, whereas the dance therapy is not about the skills, techniques only. It might involve certain steps in the process but focus is more on expression of emotions and a process oriented approach. It is about expression of oneself through the movements. The present research is an attempt to understand the difference in the effectiveness of dance as a leisure activity and the use of dance as a therapeutic intervention in the form of Dance Movement Therapy.

CHAPTER 2

REVIEW OF LITERATURE

A literature review provides an explanation, summary and assessment of any particular area of research or theory by examining the content available in various journals, books, web resources, e-journals and other research articles from other relatable sources. Review of Literature is important in giving us an understanding about the research trends and research gap on a particular topic. While exploring a particular topic and to express to the readers how a research fits within a greater field of study the literature reviews are an important part of the research which not only provides an overview of the chosen topic but also provides important insights to the research so as to carefully plan the research, its objectives, methodology, tools etc.

2.1 Importance of Review of Literature

Any subject or area of research enters through various phases of intellectual progression by which the subjects evolves and changes as per the changing dimensions. The knowledge components in the research is updated, modified, changed, accepted or rejected due the contribution of various researches on that subject or area. Every researcher must conduct a thorough review of literature so that the research efforts can be directed towards meaningful contribution to the field of study.

Review of literature requires higher order of abilities where the researcher analyses the existing literature, synthesize the outputs of various researches to develop an understanding and also evaluates the available researches to find out an appropriate plan of action for one's own research. Review of literature is helpful in various ways to the researcher.

- The most important contribution of a review of literature is identification of the research gap on a field of study. It would not only give correct direction to the researcher but the knowledge created through the research will help in filling the existing research gap which is very much needed for the advancement of a discipline.

- The existing knowledge also need to be tested in the light of new paradigms, situations hence review of literature provides an opportunity to provide a fresh interpretation of the previous research work.
- The researcher can frame appropriate research objectives, hypotheses and can select relevant methods and sample on the basis of previous researches.
- A meta-analytic review of literature is especially useful in developing an understanding about the areas or topics where conflicting or contradictory results have been obtained.

2.2 Sources of Review of Literature

The sources of review of literature are the original articles published in both print and electronic forms. The availability of electronic databases have eased and supported the review work and has given access of worldwide researches to the aspiring researchers. Some review research papers which are based on the reviews of the reviews is also very helpful in giving a researcher a better insight on the chosen topic and is also time saving. The sources can also original written work- poem, diaries, court records, interviews, surveys and original research/fieldwork and research published in scholarly/academic journals, dictionaries, encyclopaedia, textbooks and books and articles that interpret, review or synthesize original research/fieldwork.

Indexes- provides citations that fully identify a work with information such as name of the author, titles of a book, articles or journals, publisher and publication date, volume and issue number and page number.

Abstracts- summarize the primary or secondary sources,

Databases- are original indexes that usually include abstracts for each primary or secondary resource and may also include a digital copy of the resource.

2.3 The Present Research

The present research attempts to study the effect of Dance Training and Dance Movement Therapy (DMT) on the personality and psychophysical health of an individual. The present research attempts to emphasize Dance Training/Therapy as it has been proven in different researches that dance training has potential positive effects on physical, mental and emotional well-being. Although the number of researches conducted using DMT as an intervention have been limited in India, that's why the present research will be useful in understanding the role of dance in different psychological variables in Indian context.

2.4 Review of Literature

The reviews of the previous research work have been done in different parts on the basis of dependent variables of the study. The review of literature is focused on the studies conducted on dance training and dance movement therapy and its relationship with the selected dependent variables. The present study has included Personality, Psychophysical health and Anxiety as the dependent variables; hence reviews have been presented separately for these variables. Then the studies of dance movement therapy with other variables have also been presented in the later section.

2.4.1 Research on Personality

University of Haifa, (2020) found that Dance Movement Therapy (DMT) has showed a positive response on bringing physical movements among elderly patients, It also improved quality of life and the familial ties between grandparents and grandchildren. For conducting the study, sixteen dance movement therapists met with their grandmothers for performing three free-form dance sessions. The goal behind these sessions was to determine method by which these sessions would affect each group and how the intergeneration bonds can be strengthen between them. It was seen that initially grandmothers were nervous over their ability to provide a meaningful experience but as they were instructed to see their actions in mirror, encouragement was given regarding their abilities and in between they were provided with rest when they needed, there was more involvement from their side. It was found that elderly populations can improve their physical and mental health and also more connect with their loved ones due to their involvement in dance-movement therapy.

Stephanie (2015) studied that dancers are at high danger of creating cluttered eating mentalities, prominently due to disguised slimness standards. Albeit the large five character characteristics have been demonstrated to be related with eating mentalities in day by day life, in dancers where eating issues and slenderness standards disguise could be remarkable little is thought about these affiliations and the job of the disguise of slimness standards in this relationship The examination included 180 seriously preparing dancers with a normal time of 15.6 years (SD = 2.8). Dancers finished polls estimating the huge five character attributes, disguise of slimness standards and self-guideline of eating mentalities in sport. Bootstrapped intercession examinations showed that neuroticism was contrarily connected with self-guideline of eating perspectives, both straightforwardly and by implication through the intervening job of disguised slenderness standards. This investigation recommended that: (a) neuroticism is a weakness factor for self-guideline of eating perspectives in dancers, as effectively confirmed in everyone, and (b) the disguise of slenderness standards is a pathway through which neuroticism influences self-guideline of eating mentalities. The large five model is along these lines mostly identified with the disguise of slenderness standards and eating mentalities in dancers.

Dinesha & Simpson (2014) studied the relationship between dance movement classes and disruptive behaviour on a sample of 45 at risk students in an urban high school setting. The findings supported the hypothesis that a) dance classes can be utilized as an intervention to reduce stress and b) students who participate in dance programs in public school settings will develop self-control, self-regulation and exhibit less disruptive behaviour.

Alexandros et al. (2012) studied that youth who were involved in dance. The different images were shown on studies regarding effects of dance practices. Most of them referred that dance promotes their personal opportunities, increased levels of socialisation and characteristic behaviour among its participants. The level of socialisation differs according to dance forms and it is also seen that person involves in dance benefitted not only in childhood and adolescence but also were benefitted in adulthood and mature age. The aim of the present review was to provide an overview of major findings of studies concerning the social-physiological outcomes of dance practices, in a general population as well as for adults and adolescents. The typical personality profiles of dancers depended upon the dance form of dancers were relatively high on emotionality strong achievement motivated and exhibits less favourably self-attitudes. Outcomes of dance therapy revealed that better understanding of the true nature of social-psychological outcomes can be provided if specific influential factors are taken into consideration. (i.e.,participants, characteristics, type of guidance, social context and structural qualities of the dance)

Amber & Lynn (2011), studied that individual dance movement therapy is introduced as a modality for healing the wounds of torture. The impact of torture on the body, the self, and relationships, and how this can affect treatment using individual dance movement therapy, was addressed. The author concluded that dance movement therapy, following the experience of torture, can be beneficial in rebuilding an individual's sense of wholeness and self, and in improving interaction skills and relationship capacity.

Shawna (2010) did a theoretical synthesis combining the concepts from Chadian dance/movement therapy and the Responsive Classroom approach to teaching and learning, and suggested a proactive behavioural management style for dance/ movement therapists that incorporated aspects from these two frameworks. For this synthesis, Chadian dance/movement therapy and Responsive Classroom techniques were adapted and implemented. Through combining these two methods, the researcher suggested a unique treatment model as a way to prevent and confront violent and aggressive behaviours of children that were present in a dance/movement therapy session.

Sarah et al. (2006) studied the impact of physical activity on body image dissatisfaction and physical self-perceptions. The research investigated the effects of 6-week aerobic dance on these variables with 50 British schoolgirls aged 13–14 years. A cross-over design was used with two equivalent groups taught normal physical education and aerobic dance in a different order. The Body Attitude Questionnaire (BAQ) and Children and Youth Physical Self-Perception Profile (CY-PSPP) were administered as pre, mid and post-test to each participant in each group before the first intervention, at the changeover and after 12 weeks. The results of this study revealed that participation in 6 weeks of aerobic dance significantly reduced body image dissatisfaction (Attractiveness, Feeling Fat, Salience and Strength and Fitness) and enhanced physical self-perceptions (Body Attractiveness and Physical Self-Worth), although these improvements were not sustained. The implications and future research directions are discussed.

Gronlund & Renck & Weibull (2005) studied a short-term dance movement therapy (DMT) for two young boys with symptoms related to Attention Deficit Hyperactivity Disorder (ADHD). The aim was to investigate the effect and value of DMT as an alternative treatment and to describe the process. The DMT lasted ten sessions and took place once a week during three months. In a case study multiple data sources were used to triangulate the data and describe the DMT process. The DMT has promoted a positive change to a certain extent. DMT provided in paired groups for a minimum of ten weeks will (1) improve the motor function and (2) reduce the behavioural and emotional symptoms of boys aged 5–7 diagnosed with ADHD.

Koshland & Wittaker (2004) examined a 12-week dance movement therapy-based violence prevention program with 54 multicultural elementary school children, and found that it was effective in reducing aggressive behaviours. The program used a dance movement therapy group process that focused on socialization and engagement of children in creative, problem solving experiences. Data showed a decrease in the number of aggressive incidents reported to the principal for the entire school, the decrease in number of incidents for participating classrooms was greater than that for those that did not participate.

Judge et al. (2002) stated that their study reports results of a meta-analysis linking traits from the 5-factor model of personality to overall job satisfaction. Using the model as an organizing framework, 334 correlations from 163 independent samples were classified according to the model. The estimated true score correlations with job satisfaction were -.29 for Neuroticism, .25 for Extraversion, .02 for Openness to Experience, .17 for Agreeableness, and .26 for Conscientiousness. Results further indicated that only the relations of Neuroticism and Extraversion with job satisfaction generalized across studies. As a set, the Big Five traits had a multiple correlation of .41 with job satisfaction, indicating support for the validity of the dispositional source of job satisfaction when traits are organized according to the 5-factor model.

Fern & Meg (1991) studied that dance movement therapy can make to the treatment of battered women. By motivating female victims of domestic violence to act, dance movement therapy addresses patterns of helplessness, ambivalence, and inactivity. Dance movement interventions help women internalize a positive self-concept as well as gain physical and emotional control. In keeping with the short-term, crisis-oriented nature of standard treatment of battered women, a psychosocial plan of intervention which addresses their isolation and immobilization is recommended.

Crain et al. (1983) studied that Educable Mentally Retarded (EMR) adolescents may exhibit problems in social and physical development in comparison with their normal peers. The purpose of this investigation was to study the effects of a 10-week dance program on EMR adolescents. A multiple measurement approach was employed to assess potential effects. Results suggested that nature of participation, consistency of participation, and the design of the curriculum are factors that affect the improvement of social and physical behaviours such as cooperation, dance skills, increased movement repertoire, rhythms, leadership and successful peer teaching.

2.4.2 Research on Anxiety

Vicky et al. (2019) studied that three hundred and fifty-one people with depression (mild to severe) participated, 192 of whom attended DMT groups while receiving treatment as usual (TAU) and 159 received TAU only. Qualitative findings suggest there was a decrease in depression scores in favour of DMT groups in all studies. Subgroup analysis performed on depression scores before and 3 months after the completion of DMT groups suggested changes in favour of the DMT groups. When sensitivity analysis was performed, RCTs at high risk of bias were excluded, leaving only studies with adult clients up to the age of 65. In these studies, the highest effect size was found favouring DMT plus TAU for adults with depression, when compared to TAU only.

Sabine et al.(2019) analysed the intervention of DMT and found that DMT was a significant moderator of results by means of sensitivity analysis. Results thus observed showed that DMT proved to be beneficial in reduction of depression, anxiety and increases quality of life and interpersonal and cognitive skills and the dance interventions shows increase in (psycho) motor skills. Larger effects sizes outcomes from the observational measures might be the reasons behind indicating bias whereas most of the effects remained stable or slightly increased in the follow up data obtained post 22 weeks of the intervention.

Mastura et al. (2015) studied the effect of a 12-week low intensity dance exercise intervention in the treatment of hostility subscale, anxiety subscale and depression subscale among overweight women working in Malaysia in an attempt of Sports for all. It was concluded that low intensity dance therapy exercise intervention of "Aero mass" had contributed greatly to the positive findings concerning physical health and psychological well-being among overweight women in Malaysia.

Sabine et al. (2014), in their studies evaluated the effectiveness of dance movement therapy (DMT) and the therapeutic use of dance for the treatment of health-related psychological problems. Results suggested that DMT and dance are effective for increasing quality of life and decreasing clinical symptoms such as depression and anxiety. Positive effects were also found on the increase of subjective well-being, positive mood, affect, and body image.

Pinniger et al. (2013) observed that DMT and dance are useful in increasing quality of life and also there is decrease in clinical symptoms such as depression and anxiety also there is increase in positive effects is seen an increase of subjective wellbeing, positive mood and body image. The 8 week program was conducted in which 64 participants were assessed before and after 1 month follow up programme was conducted. In this programme the dependent variables like depression, anxiety, stress, fatigue and insomnia and their symptoms were measured. Positive psychology measures were also measured for self-efficacy, satisfaction with life and mindfulness. The scores thus observed were recorded on the control group basis which is discussed here. Group of participants having depression, stress and was not satisfied with life showed benefits by meditation. In the same way participants of exercise group showed decreased depression but the self-efficacy was persistent at post test and the stress was significant at follow up. At post follow-up participants of Tango group had also shown decrease in depression and insomnia and increase in life satisfaction and mindfulness.

Andrea & Karkou & Meekums (2012) studied that depression affects 121 million people worldwide (WHO, 2010). The socio-economic repercussions of depression are putting an enormous strain on UK and US governmental health budgets. Regarding treatment interventions, Dance Movement Therapy and other arts therapies are widely practiced around the world as a treatment of choice for depression. Research evidence suggested that exercise has positive effects on mood. Similarly, it has been argued that dance has a positive social-cultural influence on a person's wellbeing.

Marjolein & Van der (2011), studied that mood can influence our everyday behaviour and people often seek to reinforce, or to alter their mood, for example by turning on music. Music listening while driving is a popular activity. However, little is known about the impact of music listening while driving on physiological state and driving performance. In the present experiment, it was investigated whether individually selected music can induce mood and maintain moods during a simulated drive. In addition, effects of positive, negative, and no music on driving behaviour and physiological measures were assessed for normal and high cognitive demanding rides. Subjective mood ratings indicated that music successfully maintained mood while driving. Narrow lane width drives increased task demand as shown in effort ratings and increased swerving. Furthermore, respiration rate was lower during music listening compared to rides without music, while no effects of music were found on heart rate. Overall, the current study demonstrates that music listening in car influences the experienced mood while driving, which in turn can impact driving behaviour.

Pericleous & Isabella (2011), in his study he focused on the effects of dance movement therapy on people with depression. However, the results have pointed in a positive direction. He believed that if movement therapists as well as psychotherapists pay close attention to this condition, there will be a significant increase in research on using dance to reduce severe depression and melancholia.

Jaclyn (2010) studied the effects of dance therapy and relaxation therapy on anxiety level in college students, 24 undergraduate students from Catholic Liberal Arts College in New England were selected as participants and categorised into two groups. The first group was provided with dance therapy treatment in which students followed an instructor via videotape so to reduce their anxiousness level and the other group was provided with relaxation therapy treatment in which students listened to audio tape which is composed of music that tense and relax muscle group accompanied with deep breathing. The outcome of the study has showed that dance therapy experienced greater decrease in anxiety levels due to processes of self-expression and nonverbal communication which helps students to release their feeling of anxiousness. All students were administered with the Speilberger State-Trait Anxiety Inventory.

Sabine et al. (2007) studied the specific effects of a dance intervention on the decrease of depression and the increase of vitality and positive affect in 31 psychiatric patients with main or additional diagnosis of depression. Patients participated in one of three conditions: a dance group performing a traditional upbeat circle dance, a group that listened just to the music of the dance (music only), and a group that moved on a home trainer bike (ergometer) up to the same level of arousal as the dance group (movement only). While all three conditions alleviated or stabilized the condition of the patients, results suggest that patients in the dance group profited most from the intervention. They showed significantly less depression than participants in the music group ($p < .001$) and in the ergometer group ($p < .05$), and more vitality (p

< .05) than participants in the music group on post-test self-report scales immediately after the intervention. Stimulating circle dances can thus have a positive effect on patients with depression and may be recommended for use in dance/movement therapy and other complementary therapies.

Koch & Morlinghaus & Fuchs (2007) conducted an study on 31 patients with main or additional depression and have shown decrease of depression and increase in vitality and positive effects due to the dance intervention. Patients who participated in any of these three groups out of these groups one was performing traditional dance upbeat in circle manner, second group only listened music (not danced) and third who moved to home on home trainer bike (ergo meter) were aroused to same level as that of dance group (movement only). Results of study indicates that the patients in the group of dance movement were benefitted the most by the intervention as they showed significant reduction in depression in comparison to the patients of music group ($p>.001$) and to that of patient of ergo meter ($p >.05$) and more vitality ($p >.05$) than participants in music group on post-test, self-report immediately after the intervention. These led to the outcome that simulating circle dance can be recommended for use in dance/movement therapy and other complimentary therapies as it shows positive effects on the patients of depression.

Jeong et al. (2005) provided a 12-week Dance Movement Therapy (DMT) program and then assessed the profiles of psychological health and changes in neurohormones of adolescents with mild depression The outcomes has showed that DMT can help in stabilising sympathetic nervous system and it was also seen that DMT can be effective in beneficially modulating concentration of serotonin and dopamine and can improve physiological distress in adolescents with mild depression.

Andre L.& John R. (1990) studied that the effects of modern dance on anxiety. While using the Spielberg State-Trait Anxiety Inventory, state anxiety was assessed before and after 3-month education programme. A class in modern dance was followed by the target group. Three categories of control group are constituted i.e. (1) physical group to control for the effects of exercise. (2). music group to control for aesthetic sensitivity training and (3) a mathematical group. Many factors like age, sex, attitude towards dance and previous experience in dance, sport and relaxation were measured and it is seen that dance therapy reduces anxiety while control activities were unable to do so. On examining concomitant variables, it was concluded that the result could not be accounted for by any obvious artefacts.

2.4.3 Research on Psychophysical Health

Young et al. (2016) studied that dancing is characterised by physical movement in accordance with rhythm perception. Twelve sport dancers and 12 age- and sex-matched young adults who had no dance experience (control group) were recruited. Body intelligence and brain activity were assessed in both groups using the Body Intelligence Scale (BIS) and resting state functional magnetic resonance imaging. BIS scores of dancers were higher than those of control subjects. The dancer group showed increased functional connectivity from the precentral gyrus to the right cingulate gyrus, right occipital fusiform gyrus, right inferior frontal gyrus, right medial frontal gyrus, left inferior frontal gyrus, right parietal postcentral gyrus, and right frontal lobe compared with control subjects. Sport dancers had increased body intelligence sensitivity compared with matched controls. In addition, the characteristics of dance, including physical movement in accordance with rhythm perception, might be associated with increased brain activity in the somato-sensory and rhythm perception networks.

Orsolya et al. (2015) studied that dancing is a popular form of physical exercise and studies have shown that dancing can decrease anxiety, increase self-esteem, and improve psychological wellbeing. The aim of the current study was to explore the motivational basis of recreational social dancing and develop a new psychometric instrument to assess dancing motivation. The sample comprised 447 salsa and/or ballroom dancers (68% female; mean age 32.8 years) who completed an online survey. Eight motivational factors were identified via exploratory factor analysis and comprise a new Dance Motivation Inventory: Fitness, Mood Enhancement, Intimacy, Socialising, Trance, Mastery, Self-confidence and Escapism. Mood Enhancement was the strongest motivational factor for both males and females, although motives differed according to gender. Dancing intensity was predicted by three motivational factors: Mood Enhancement, Socialising, and Escapism. The eight dimensions identified cover possible motives for social recreational dancing, and the DMI proved to be a suitable measurement tool to assess these motives. The explored motives such as Mood Enhancement, Socialising and Escapism appear to be similar to those identified in other forms of behaviour such as drinking alcohol, exercise, gambling, and gaming.

Falisha et al. (2015) studied that dance is a universal form of human expression that offers a rich source for scientific study. Dance provides a unique opportunity to investigate brain plasticity and its interaction with behaviour. Several studies have investigated the behavioural correlates of dance, but less is known about the brain basis of dance. Studies on dance observation suggested that long- and short-term dance training affect brain activity in the action observation and simulation networks. Despite methodological challenges, the feasibility of conducting neuro-imaging while dancing has been demonstrated, and several brain regions have been implicated in dance execution. It was suggested that long-term dance training changes both gray and white matter structure. This article provided a critical summary of work investigating the neural correlates of dance.

Laura et al. (2015) investigated how episodic memory performance can be improved by manipulating the factors that are crucial for successful encoding. There is an ongoing debate about whether a complex stimulus such as music can improve memory, and in particular memory for words, rather than interfere with correct encoding of information. This study aimed to investigate whether verbal episodic memory can be improved by background context of instrumental music. Twenty young adults were asked to memorize different lists of words presented against a background of music, environmental sounds or silence. Their episodic memory performance was then tested in terms of item and source memory scores. Results revealed better memory performance under the music condition than with environmental sounds or silence in the retrieval of the context (i.e. source) of the encoded material. These findings, contrasting with studies showing an interfering effect of music, are discussed in terms of both methodological and theoretical perspectives with the aim of furthering the debate about music and memory. In sum, our results indicate that music can specifically act as a facilitating encoding context for verbal episodic memory, opening important perspectives for music as a rehabilitation tool for episodic memory deficits.

Duim do Nascimento & Silva (2015) studied the functional rehabilitation after a fall involving motor and proprioceptive work as well as being closely connected with psycho-emotional aspects. Dance movement therapy is kind of creative exercise which utilises body in developing this art. After considering studies on dance movement therapy they perform the quasi-experimental study in ten elderly patients for rehabilitation and then they were evaluated on the basis of their quality of life (WHOQOL-Bref), balance (Tinetti Balance Scale- BBS and Berg scale) and mobility (Timed "Up and Go" test-TUG), before and after treatment. Total 16 sessions of therapies was conducted with the goal of creating body self-awareness, spatial perception, co-ordination in relation to song and movement and creativity. Improvement in quality of life has been shown by student's t-test (physical p=0.028, psychological p=0.049, Social p=0.027 and environmental p=0.032). In the same way improvement is seen in balance and mobility with the help of Wilcoxon test (BBS p=0.016; Berg Scale p=0.017, TUG p=0.005). The outcome of the study has supported the theory that dance has positive effect on motor aspects which results in improving mobility and balance and on practicing regularly dance movement therapy in group it can improve quality of life. This study postulates that DMT is beneficial and also low-cost therapy for elderly women who has a history of fall.

Arpita C. (2013) studied that Dance increases total body movement, which helps to improve circulatory, respiratory, skeletal and muscular systems. It has a positive effect on physical health as well as mental and emotional wellbeing. In western world, dance has been used as a form of therapy in many hospitals and medical settings, whether alternate or complementary. The effects of different folk and tribal dance forms of West Bengal on physical, mental and social health are discussed in her study.

Harvard Medical School Department of Neurobiology (2012) studied that the Latin-style dance program known as Zumba improves mood and certain cognitive skills, such as visual recognition and decision-making. Other studies show that dance helps reduce stress, increases levels of the feel-good hormone serotonin, and helps develop new neural connections, especially in regions involved in executive function, long-term memory, and spatial recognition.

Raquel & de (2010) In patients with Multiple Sclerosis (MS) balance and motor coordination within a physiotherapy program when dance was used as therapeutic resource also the patients aided with dance intervention shows the positive effect in neurological function scales (EDSS, NRS, MDS) as they achieved greater postural and balance control. The patient also reported an amelioration of her emotional state. This patient started to perform his previously daily life activities as there was improved physical functioning.

Asmita (2010), Cognitive development is positively affected by the factors of dance therapy which is proven through the result that dance movement therapy create good environment for cognitive development. It is seen that it can be beneficial to the most of the children and can also be implied to maximum number of teachers.

Eva (2004) examined comparative changes in hormonal, emotional, physical and visual status changes in female fibromyalgia (FMS) patients after treatment with Creative Art therapy; dance/movement therapy in comparison with controls. Patients with FMS disorder suffers for chronic pain and the reason behind are musculoskeletal aches, stiffness and pain where perturbations in the stress-axis and high scores on somatic anxiety and muscular tensions also have been found. In this study 36 female FMS patients are included and then divided in two groups which are treatment group and control group. Concentration of hormones in plasma like prolactin, dehydroepiandrostone sulphate (DHEA-S), cortisol and neuropeptide Y (NPY) and of cortisol in saliva were taken and then analysed. Different verbal self-rating scales concerning well-being pain, personality and life events among other things have been used. Patients with FMS syndrome who are affected by video-viewing were assessed and then they were evaluated together with interviews regarding self-perception phenomenon of video viewing (a phenomenal hermeneutic method). It is seen that patients after going through dance/ movement therapy has shown improvement in both psychological and physical functions which is proven by visual analysis. The video interpretation technique (VIT) and self-figure drawing captured treatment that were not evident from verbal scales or reflected in hormonal levels. Biological markers may take longer treatment period to activate the HPA axis and its inter-related hormones and peptides.

McCord, Nichols & Patterson (1989) studied the effects of a 12-week program of low impact aerobic dance conditioning on VO2max, submaximal heart rates and body composition of college-aged women. Sixteen women exercised three times per week for approximately 45 minutes per session at 75-85% of their heart rate reserve. VO2max was measured by indirect calorimetry using a treadmill protocol. Submaximal heart rates were measured by electrocardiography, and body fat was assessed by hydrostatic weight. All testing was conducted within one week pre- and post-training. Training sessions consisted of a 5-10 minute warm up, 30-35 minute low impact aerobic dance segment and a 5 minute cool down. Posttest results revealed a small (7%), but significant increase in VO2max (pre: 38.3 ml/kg/min; post: 41.3 ml/kg/min, X +/- SD, p less than 0.05). Submaximal heart rates at minutes 2-3, 3-4 and 4-5 of the graded exercise test decreased significantly. Body fat decreased from 25 +/- 6.8% to 21 +/- 6.3% (p less than 0.01) with no post training change in body weight. It was concluded that low impact aerobic dance is as effective as other endurance training regimens in improving cardiovascular fitness and decreasing body fat.

2.4.4 Research on dance with other variables

Jordan & Donahue (2020) studied subjective strategies to investigate the encounters of National Grid linemen for the reasons for making a dance development treatment warm-up. Data was accumulated through singular gatherings, where inquiries concerning member's physical, mental and enthusiastic wellbeing were examined comparable to their particular occupation. From the data accumulated, six topics were recognized. To address the perceived issues, eight proposed warm-ups were made. The warm ups, explicitly made from member's firsthand records, are established in both Laban Movement Analysis standards and Bartineff Fundamentals. Meetings are planned to be controlled by an authorized dance development specialist toward the start of every workday and would keep going for roughly 15 minutes. Future ramifications incorporate further exploration, which would investigate the viability and saw advantages of made meetings with line laborers to additionally investigate the advantages of dance movement treatment with the individuals who contain this dedicated population.

Elizabeth (2016) explored methods for bringing dance history directly into the studio. She showed how the movement components that have proven successful in introductory courses can be extended to in-depth studies of dance history with dancers who have formal training. Through the example of a research project on the early work of George Balanchine, it shows how kinaesthetic learners can be introduced to the scholarly side of this art form in a way that shows them its relevance and gives them tools that they can use in their own careers as dancers and choreographers. Finally, she demonstrated how this method allows students the opportunity to explore history through movement in conjunction with archival material, photographs, books, papers and videos.

Hannah et al. (2015) studied that in both partnered Latin dance and non-partnered Latin-themed aerobic dance has increased in recent years, likely a result of the gaining popularity of these types of instructor-led group classes among the mainstream dance and fitness audiences; however, the efficacy of these activities for the purposes of health promotion currently remains unclear. The purpose of this study was to simultaneously assess the physiological responses and psychological experiences during salsa dance and Zumba fitness in a community sample of physically inactive women.

Imogen & Rachel (2015) studied dancers' motivation to work in an independent capacity, and the extent to which dancers' psychological characteristics and skills enabled them to navigate a career in this demanding sector. In-depth semi-structured interviews were conducted with 14 dancers at different stages of their careers. Interviews were transcribed verbatim and content analysed. Analysis revealed that the dancers were intrinsically motivated and highly committed to the profession. Working in the independent sector offered dancers opportunities for growth and fulfilment; they appreciated the autonomy, flexibility and freedom that the independent career afforded, as well as working with new people across roles and disciplines. In order to overcome the various challenges associated with the independent role, optimism, self-belief, social support, and career management skills were crucial. The mental skills reported by the participants had developed gradually in response to the demands that they faced. Therefore, mental skills training could be invaluable for dancers to help them successfully negotiate the independent sector.

Iris (2014) studied that the more than 65 age bunch is continually expanding in size. Asset situated treatment approaches, for example, dance movement treatment (DMT) is getting more significant as they protect the poise of the older, regard their individual requirements and improve social investment. A global web-based study was shipped off 683 DMT partners, of which 113 professionals from Austria, Germany and Switzerland reacted to the accompanying inquiries: To what degree can more established individuals' advantage through DMT? What subjects arise in the meetings? Which restorative intercessions are applied? What are the proposals as to working conditions and the qualities and adapting techniques of specialists? The subjective information investigation uncovers that professionals concur that DMT improves the personal satisfaction of old individuals, encourages support of their connections and extends their assets and cooperation in exercises. The outcomes help us in planning explicit intercession suggestions.

Ho & Rainbow (2014) examined that Breast cancer patients undergoing radiotherapy often suffer from various disease symptoms such as fatigue, pain, and sleep disturbance. These symptoms have been shown to be detrimental to their daily functioning and illness prognosis. The present study aimed to examine the effects of dance movement therapy as an integrated therapeutic intervention on the disease symptoms in breast cancer patients undergoing radiotherapy. The results suggested that dance movement psychotherapy may have therapeutic effects in reducing the pain severity of breast cancer patients receiving radiotherapy.

Iris (2012) conducted a study in which the intervention on quality of life was examined on the basis of the treatment outcome ten weeks dance movement therapy. This whole study was done with design of pre-test, post-test and six month follow up. 162 participants were identified and selected who are suffering from stress were randomly selected and then they were provided with movement therapy treatment group (TG) (n=97) or with wait-listed control group (WG) (65). The significant improvement was seen in psychological domain, social relations, global health, physical health and general life while in long term dance movement therapy shows great improvement in the psychological domain, spirituality and general which leads to draw the conclusion that dance movement therapy is beneficial in short as well as long term in improving quality of life.

Kiepe & Stockigt & Kiel (2012) conducted a study that dance movement therapy has a positive impact for patients with breast cancer, improving quality of life, shoulder range of motion and body image. In patients with depression psychological distress was reduced by dance therapy. Ballroom dance improved balance and coordination in patients with Parkinson's disease and disease-specific quality of life in patients with heart failure. Dance movement therapy and ballroom dance seem beneficial for patients with breast cancer, depression, Parkinson's disease, diabetes and heart failure.

Michelle (2010) considered what movement therapist does and how their administrations connect with traditional psychotherapy. The motivation behind this venture was to give data about dance movement treatment as an approach to advance the training and move towards overcoming any issues between this elective treatment and standard psychotherapies. This exploratory and spellbinding examination was brought out through semi-organized meetings. The sample (N=9) was made of up dance movement specialist who were ensured by the American Dance Therapy Association. Questions were intended to accumulate data about members segment, preparing and accreditation cycle, strategies and meaning of dance development treatment, customer qualities and building client base and report. A substance examination of discoveries showed that dance movement specialist does encounter challenges in building up an affinity inside the psychological well-being field. It was likewise found that the vast majority have a helpless comprehension of what dance movement treatment is and how it functions as psychotherapeutic treatment. Social and profound ramifications are inspected too, as they identify with the elective act of dance development treatment.

Emily (2010), This qualitative research explored creative movement processes such as dance movement therapy (DMT), authentic movement (AM), and creative dance (CD) as possible tools for transforming sexual trauma for women. Eleven movement professionals were interviewed in a semi-structured research format. Her direct experience and knowledge of sexual abuse, sexual trauma, and creative movement processes were interwoven with the research question: Do creative dance movement therapy processes contribute to the dynamic of healing for women transforming sexual trauma? These findings were inconclusive for the greater population of survivors of sexual abuse and sexual trauma. However, there were indications that DMT, AM, and CD may be potential tools for recovery. This research contributed to a dialogue about sexual abuse and recovery from sexual trauma.

Than et al. (2010)A nonpharmacological method can be an alternative or complement to analgesics. The aim of this study was to evaluate if music medicine influences pain and anxiety in children undergoing lumbar punctures. A randomized clinical trial was used in 40 children (aged 7-12 years) with leukaemia, followed by interviews in 20 of these participants. The participants were randomly assigned to a music group (n = 20) or control group (n = 20). The primary outcome was pain scores and the secondary was heart rate, blood pressure, respiratory rate, and oxygen saturation measured before, during, and after the procedure. Anxiety scores were measured before and after the procedure. Interviews with open-ended questions were conducted in conjunction with the completed procedures. The results showed lower pain scores and heart and respiratory rates in the music group during and after the lumbar puncture. The anxiety scores were lower in the music group both before and after the procedure. The findings from the interviews confirmed the quantity results through descriptions of a positive experience by the children, including less pain and fear.

Tomas et al. (2010) studied that the relationship between individual differences and specific uses of music, referring to why and how people use music in everyday life. Questionnaire data from 341 respondents showed that open and intellectually engaged individuals, and those with higher IQ scores, tended to use music in a rational/cognitive way, while neurotic, introverted and non-conscientious individuals were all more likely to use music for emotional regulation (e.g. change or enhance moods). Results suggest that individual differences in personality and cognitive ability may partly determine the way in which we experience music. Limitations and suggestions for future studies are discussed

Wiley (2008) reported that the British Government had taken initiatives to include dance in promoting social and educational inclusion through arts on the basis of the results of the researches which had shown the relationship between the social classes of peoples. On analysing data it was seen that attitudes to aspects of dance varies with social class and that there was interaction between gender and social class in just one instance. The major outcome of the study was that the maximum number of children in schools should be benefited by the dance arts and also young people can have reach to aesthetic experiences that have potential to improve quality of life. It was concluded that the current limited provision within the national curriculum may be contributing to the social and educational exclusions of some pupils.

Watson & Dr Garrett (2006) of the University of Hertfordshire compared members of the Royal Ballet with a squad of British national and international swimmers. In their research, they found that the dancers scored higher than the swimmers in seven out of ten areas of fitness.

Marika & Samantha (2000) investigated the relationship between amount of exercise and psychological well-being in a broadly based sample. A questionnaire assessing amount of exercise, reasons for exercise, body satisfaction, and self-esteem was completed by 252 participants between the ages of 16 and 60 years. Participants were divided into four groups on the basis of gender and age, resulting in 70 young women, 48 young men, 73 mature women, and 61 mature men. Significant negative relationships between amount of exercise and body satisfaction and self-esteem were found for young women, and positive relationships for the remainder of the sample. Women exercised more for reasons of weight control, tone, and mood enhancement than men. For the whole sample, the first two of these reasons were associated with lower body satisfaction, while exercising for health and fitness reasons was associated with increased self-esteem. It was concluded that reasons for exercising did not provide an adequate explanation for the obtained difference in correlations across gender and age.

2.4.5 Synthesizing Reviews

The above review of literature has shown that the effect of dance and dance movement therapy has been studied on the variety of sample. The chosen sample in these researches has included the elderly population, children undergoing lumbar punctures, women who have experienced sexual trauma, dance movement specialist, patients with breast cancer, adolescents and adults who were suffering from stress, female with fibromyalgia, the patients who have Multiple Sclerosis (MS), the individuals who were undergoing functional rehabilitation after a fall, salsa and/or ballroom dancers, patients with anxiety and depression, Educable Mentally Retarded (EMR) persons and the female victims of domestic violence etc.

Dance movement therapy and dance training has been found to be effective for healing the wounds of torture, in reducing aggressive behaviours among elementary school children, in controlling the symptoms of depression and other mood disorders, in improving the physical fitness, in controlling the behavioural and emotional symptoms shown by the patients diagnosed with ADHD. It has also been found effective in developing self-control, self-regulation and in exhibiting less disruptive behaviour among at risk students. Some researchers have focused on the specific dance forms such as Zumba, Salsa and Ballroom dance etc.

2.5 Research Gap

On the basis of the above review of literature, some major **research gaps** have been identified in the proposed field of investigation.

There are fewer researches which has compared the psychological profiles of dancers and non-dancers. There are researches conducted on various samples as discussed above, the researchers comparing the adolescents on the basis of their involvement in dance training is missing.

It is also missing whether the usual dance training, which focuses on the steps, skills, acts, performance differs, differs from the therapeutic use of dance. The comparison of dance trainees and non-dance trainees and using the dance movement therapy as an intervention in the same research are also missing.

Various studies have been conducted on psychological and physical factors of dance movement therapy like effect of DMT on Depression, Cancer, Dementia, Autism but only few empirical studies are available which have studied the personality traits of dancers and how the personality traits of dancers differ from non-dancers. The present research has chosen to study the big five personality traits among dancer and then compare these personality traits with non-dancers.

Both Physical and Mental health has been an important facet of an individual's quality of life; hence present research has included psychophysical health as a variables in the study. Empirical studies on psychological and physical health related to Dance Movement Therapy in India are very few

The researches focusing the effect of DMT on anxiety in Indian contests are available but are limited in number to develop a comprehensive picture. Such researches are scantily found in the geographical area chosen for the study.

CHAPTER - 3

METHOD AND PROCEDURE

Research methodology consists of the plan, structure and the strategy a researcher adopts for conducting a research. It is important for a research to come up with the findings that are applicable on the larger groups, the intended population. Research techniques and methods are important in accuracy of the outcomes we get from the research. The techniques and system are viewed as the foundation of any exploration. This chapter gives a detailed view of the methods, tools and techniques used by the researcher

The researcher outlines research goals keeping in view the information and knowledge that one has accomplished during the time spent studying the current writings on the subject selected for the research. Survey of Literature is additionally valuable for selecting an appropriate topic for the exploration. Based on these bits of knowledge, the researcher chooses strategies from among the accessible alternatives.The researcher readies the research framework and plan, how the sample would be chosen, which techniques would be utilized for choosing test, which factors would be chosen for study, which information assortments strategies and instruments would be generally fitting for the chosen factors, what might be the scoring systems, how the information would be investigated with proper insights according to the idea of the information and so on.

Thus, it tends to be said as characterized by different analysts that methodology relates to the arrangement, structure and technique planned in order to get answer to the research questions. It also identified the control factors and makes appropriate plan to control these factors so that the precise relationships for the targeted variables can be understood and the effect of extraneous variables can be controlled. The methodology incorporates a total layout of what the researcher did from composing the speculations and their operational ramifications to the last investigation of the information.

3.1 OBJECTIVES

The title of the present research is 'Personality & Psychophysical Health in relation to Dance Training: A Therapeutic Intervention of Dance Movement Therapy'. After conducting an extensive review of literature, the following research objectives and hypotheses were framed:

1. To study the effect of Dance Training on personality (Openness, Conscientiousness, Extraversion, Agreeableness and Neuroticism), level of anxiety & psychophysical health
2. To study the effect of gender on an individual's personality, level of anxiety & psychophysical health
3. To study the interaction effect of gender (male & female) and dance training (dance trainee & non dance trainee) on personality, level of anxiety & psychophysical health
4. To prepare an intervention model based on Dance Movement Therapy
5. Therapeutic intervention of Dance Movement Therapy to study its effect on personality, level of anxiety & psychophysical health

3.2 HYPOTHESES

1. There is no difference between the personality of Dance Trainee and Non-Dance Trainee.
2. There is no difference between the psychophysical health of Dance Trainee and Non-Dance Trainee.
3. There is no difference between the level of anxiety of Dance Trainee and Non-Dance Trainee.
4. There is no difference between the personality of Males and Females.
5. There is no difference between the psychophysical health of Males and Females.
6. There is no difference between the level of anxiety of Males and Females.
7. There is no effect of therapeutic use of dance movement therapy on personality, psychophysical health and anxiety.

3.3 VARIABLES

Dance Training and Gender have been selected as the independent variables for the present research. Dance Training has two categories Dance Trainee and Non-Dance Trainee. Gender also has two categories Male and Female.

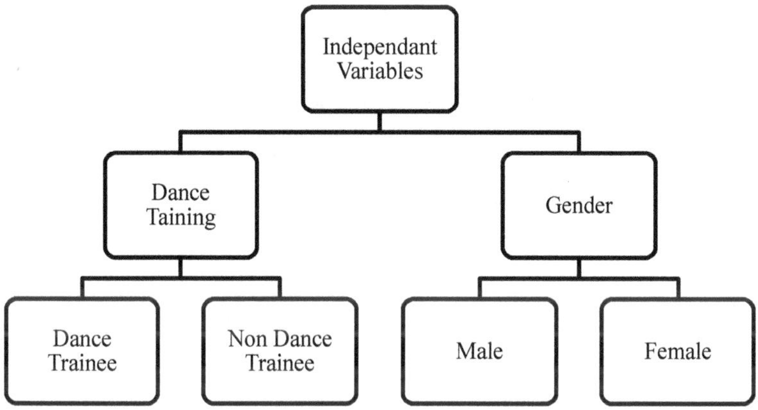

The following three variables were selected as dependents variables for the present research.

a. Personality – Big five traits

(Openness, Conscientiousness, Extraversion, Agreeableness and Neuroticism)

b. Psychophysical Health (Mental and Physical health)

c. Anxiety

3.4 RESEARCH DESIGN

The present research was conducted in two phases. In the first phase, the research collected data from the sample of 120 adolescents selected as per the factorial design shown below. In the second phase, the research conducted dance-movement therapy on 20 adolescents divided in two groups; one control and one experimental group.

Phase I

A total sample of 120 adolescents was selected as per the 2x2 factorial design.

Table 3.1 : 2x2 factorial design (Phase-I)

	Dance Trainee (B_1)	**Non-Dance Trainee (B_2)**	**Total**
Male (A_1)	A_1B_1 (N=30)	A_1B_2 (N=30)	60
Female (A_2)	A_2B_1 (N=30)	A_2B_2 (N=30)	60
Total	60	60	120

There were four groups as per the factorial design.

Group 1: Male adolescents who are receiving dance training (N=30)

Group 2: Male adolescents who are NOT receiving dance training (N=30)

Group 3: Female adolescents who are receiving dance training (N=30)

Group 4: Female adolescents who are NOT receiving dance training (N=30)

Phase II

Dance Movement Therapy Intervention

An intervention model based on the dance-movement therapy principles and techniques was prepared by the researcher. The specific techniques, number of sessions, its sequence and duration were decided to finalise an intervention model. This intervention model was used by the researcher to provide dance-movement therapy to selected adolescents in Phase-II of the research.

A Before-After Two group Control-Experimental Design was used for the Phase-II therapeutic sessions. A sample of 20 adolescents was selected randomly from 60 adolescents from Phase-I. These adolescents had never received any dance training and were a part of non-dance trainee group.. Their pre-test data on Personality, Mental Health and level of Anxiety was already available.

Table 3.2: Before-After Two Groups Design (Phase II)

Group	Pre-test	Intervention	Post-test
Control Group (N=10)	• Personality • Psychophysical health • Anxiety	No Intervention	• Personality • Psychophysical health • Anxiety
Experimental Group (N=10)	• Anxiety Personality • Psychophysical health • Anxiety	Intervention (Dance Movement Therapy)	• Personality • Psychophysical health • Anxiety

The selected 20 adolescents were randomly assigned to different groups to form two groups. To assign the treatments randomly, which group would serve as the control group and which group would serve as experimental group was also decided randomly. After formation of control and experimental groups, the experimental group was provided dance-movement therapy (DMT) as per the sessions and duration specified in the intervention model prepared by the researcher. The control group was not provided dance-movement therapy.

Once the DMT intervention was complete, post-testing for anxiety, psychophysical health and personality was done to get the comparative score to analyse the effect of DMT on the three dependent variables.

3.5 SAMPLE

Locale

The locale of the present study was confined to Udaipur district of Rajasthan. The sample was selected from the different Dance Institutes of Udaipur. The sample of non-dancers is also taken from Udaipur district.

Sample

The sample comprised of 120 adolescents out of which 60 adolescents were receiving dance training and the remaining 60 adolescents have not received any dance training. The adolescents who have received dance training have been referred to as 'Dance trainees' (DT) in the present research. The adolescents who have not received any type of dance training have been referred as 'non-dance trainees' (NDT) in the present research. In each of the DT and NDT group, equal numbers of male and female adolescents were selected in the sample. That means, in each group, there were 30 male and 30 female adolescents selected as per the factorial design of the research discussed earlier. The sample was selected from different dance Institutes of Udaipur district in Rajasthan in Phase-I. In Phase-II, 20 adolescents selected randomly from non-dance trainee group of Phase-I were selected.

A list was created by including male and female learners in the age range between 18-30 years from different dance institutes of Udaipur. 30 boys and 30 girls were selected randomly from that list to be a part of 'dance trainee' group.

Inclusion criteria: In this study, adolescents of age group 18-30 years, who have undergone at least 3 months of dance training, were selected as Dance Trainees.

Exclusion criteria: Samples below the age group 18 and above the age 30 were not be included.

SAMPLING PLAN

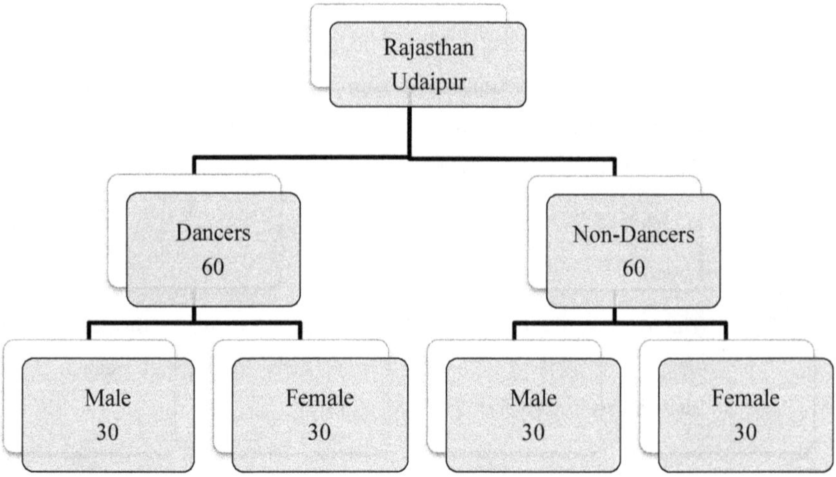

3.6 DEMOGRAPHIC PROFILE OF THE SAMPLE

The following information related to demographic factors was also collected during data collection. The respondents were asked to fill a Personal Data Sheet along with the tools used for dependent variables of the study.

- Name
- Age
- Gender
- Education
- School/College
- Marital Status
- Dance Trainee or Non-Dance Trainee
- Name of Dance Trainee Institute, if any
- Duration of dance raining

Table 3.3 : Age-wise Classification of Sample

Categories	Frequency	Percent
18-21 years	62	51.7
22-25 years	42	35.0
26-30 years	16	13.3

Table 3.4 : Education-wise Classification of the Sample

Categories	Frequency	Percent
Secondary/ Senior Secondary	14	11.7
Graduation	73	60.8
Post Graduation	33	27.5
Total	120	100.0

3.7 PSYCHOLOGICAL TESTS USED FOR DATA COLLECTION

According to Anastasi and Urbina, psychological tests involve observations made on a "carefully chosen sample of an individual's behavior. They are useful to measure unobserved constructs. The tools are an important elements of any research. The tools used in a research should be standardized so that the results obtained are more reliable. A test shall have the folowing characteristics of a Psychological test- Standardization, Objectivity, Test Norms, Reliability and Validity.

The present research attempts to study the effect of Dance Training and Dance Movement Therapy (DMT) on the personality and psychophysical well-being of an individual. The effect of Dance on Personality, Anxiety and Psychophysical health were studied. The following tools were used for collecting Data-

Table 3.4 : Psychological tests/tools used for Data Collection

Variable	Name of the Test/Scale	Author
Personality	Big Five personality test	Costa & McCrae, 1992
Anxiety	Sinha Anxiety Scale	D. N. Sinha, 1976
Psychophysical health	P.G.I. Health Questionnaire	S K Verma, 1971

3.7.1 Big Five Personality Test-

The NEO Five-Factor Inventory is used for assess personality on five dimensions i.e. are Neuroticism, Extraversion, Openness, Agreeableness, and Conscientiousness. This inventory has a number of versions like240, 180, 96 or 60 items inventory. However, the most applicable to the study carried out, is the 60 items inventory, with least number of responses, within a 5-point scale and the same is described below-

a) **Neuroticism (N)-** It means adjustment or emotional stability with maladjustment or neuroticism. It is the experience of negative feeling such as embarrassment, fear, guilt, sadness etc. High scores in Neuroticism means less able to control their impulses and unable to cope with stress. The individuals who score low on Neuroticism are emotionally stable.

b) **Extraversion (E)-** Extraversion means quantity and intensity of interpersonal interactions, activity level, need for stimulation and capacity for joy. High scores on this dimension tends to be sociable, active, talkative, person oriented, optimistic, fun loving. Low scores show personality of reserved nature, sober, un-exuberant, aloof, task oriented, retiring and quiet.

c) **Openness (O)-** This term includes proactive seeking and appreciation of experience for its own sake; toleration for and exploration of the unfamiliar. High scores on this scale are curious, having broad interests, creative, original, and imaginative. Low scores tend to be conventional, down to earth, with narrow interests, un-artistic and un-analytical.

d) **Agreeableness (A)-** how effectively you get on with different people is calculated by this dimension. High scores on this dimension indicate expected to be a soft hearted, good nurtured, trusting, helpful and forgiving. Low scores show rude, suspicious, uncooperative, irritable and manipulative.

e) **Conscientiousness (C)-** This term evaluates how a person is motivate towards his goal, the degree of his determination. High scores mean hardworking, organized, reliable, punctual, self-discipline etc. Low scores indicate aimless, unreliable, lazy, careless, negligent and hedonistic.

Scoring-

N: If scored below 13 it means low (and below 6 very low) on N and if scored above 21 it means high on N. Otherwise, scored in average range.

E: If scored below 24 (below 18 very low) it means low on E. If scored above 30 (above 36 very high) it means high on E. Otherwise scored in average range.

O: If scored 23 it means low on O (below 18 very low). Above 30 high on O (above 36 very high). Otherwise you scored in average range.

A: If you scored below 29 (below 24 very low) it means low on A. If scored above 35 it means high on A. (and above 40 very high). Otherwise scored in average range.

C: If scored below 30 it means low on C. (below 25 very low). If scored above 37 you are high on C (above 43 very high). Otherwise scored in average range.

a) Reliability- "The reliability of the NEO-FFI had been established by evaluating the Cronbach's-alpha reliability coefficients. The value of the coefficient is 0.90, 0.78, 0.76, 0.86 and 0.90 for the dimensions of neuroticism, extraversion, openness, agreeableness and conscientiousness, respectively. These values are high enough (0.76 and more) to reflect on the reliability of the inventory."

3.7.2 PGI Health Questionnaire-

Directions for Administration and Scoring-

"If the respondent can read Hindi give him/her the test sheet and a pencil. Ask him to put atick against questions he agrees with. Most of the respondents are able to finish this test within 5 minutes. The number of ticks on section A and B indicate the respective scores, which can be then added up to give a total score also.

If the respondent is illiterate, read to him/her each question slowly and record his/her response. If a respondent does not understand the question repeat it or briefly explain it. Avoid long explanations and suggestions on how to reply. Unsophisticated respondents often say things which they think are expected of them and not what they genuinely feel. This test will be useful only if one is able to record what respondent genuinely feels about himself/herself. One's own suggestions should be strictly avoided.

There is no fixed number of questions above which all neurotics should score on this test but in our studies of over 500 persons we found that if a person ticks more than 10 items, chances are high that he has got marked neurotic trends.

A high score need not always indicate neurosis, but (a) it shows a propensity to develop neurotic symptoms under stress, and (b) neurotic scores higher than normal. Some of the 'normals' do develop symptoms later and a few neurotics tend to deny the presence of symptoms which may be considered as socially undesirable responses. Use of a lie scale in addition to it, may prove useful, although the correlations with lie score of the present scale are found low."

3.7.3 Sinha Anxiety Scale-

A test was developed which could tap the different areas or dimensions as well as forms of manifestations of anxiety because manifestation of anxiety is multi-dimensional.

So, questions were drafted to bring out self-ratings on items definitive of anxiety reactions to the subsequent areas:

- Health, appearance and injury.
- Area of ambition.

- Family anxieties
- Anxieties regarding friendship and love
- Social relations and social approval
- Worries regarding the future
- Worries about civilization, war, virtue
- Guilt and shame
- Physical and physiological manifestation
- Purely psychological manifestation

The Self-Analysis form, which is a preliminary form of test, had a total of 140 items of theYes/No type.

Reliability

As determined by the Table, both split-half and test and retest methods had high reliability. It was found that the Standard error of measurement was 6.10 which shows that the true score didn't diverge way too much from the true value.

Table 3.5: Sinha Anxiety Scale Reliability

Method	N	r	Index of reliability	S. E. m.
Split-half	239	.86	.92	6.10
Test-retest	88	.73	.85	

Validity

The count on the Taylor's MAS as amended by the author, was used as the first validation criterion. Taylor's MAS was administered on all the 70 subjects who had taken the test. The correlation that was measured on the unrevised version of the scale was of the similar value as of the test which was .69 which indicated that the two tests were measuring almost the similar

3.8 PROCEDURE OF DATA COLLECTION-

3.8.1 Phase-I

Data were collected through individual face to face interaction. The data collection was done in year 2019. The data was collected at the time of the convenience of the respondents. A comfortable environment was provided to the respondents by establishing proper rapport with them. The purpose of the research was explained during the rapport building process. They were informed about the purpose of the study and their consent for participation in the study was obtained. They were ensured about the confidentiality of the information that they provided. It was also informed that the obtained information will be used only for the research purpose. The personal details like their name and other information will be kept confidential. They were also asked if they had any queries with reference to the research. The respondent's permission was obtained to start the data collection process.

The sets of Personality test, Anxiety Scale and P.G.I. health questionnaire were given to them one by one. They were also instructed to fill their personal information sheet on the front page. The instructions used specifically for various tests and tools used in the research have been given below.

Instructions of the Big-five Personality Test-

"Write only where indicated in this item booklet. Carefully read all of the instructions before beginning. This questionnaire contains 60 statements. Read each statement carefully. For each statement, fill in the circle with the response that best represents your opinion. Make sure that your answer is in the correct box.

Fill in SD if you strongly disagree or the statement is definitely false.

Fill in D if you disagree or the statement is mostly false.

Fill in N if you are neutral on the statement, if you cannot decide, or if the statement is about equally true and false.

Fill in A if you agree or the statement is mostly true.

Fill in SA if you strongly agree or the statement is definitely true.

Note that the responses are numbered in rows.

Fill in only one response for each statement. Respond to all of the statement, making sure that you fill in the correct response. DO NOT ERASE! If you need to change an answer, make an X through the incorrect response and then fill in the correct response.

Before responding to the statement, turn to the inside of this Item Booklet and enter your name, age, sex, ID number (if any) and today's date."

Instructions of Sinha Anxiety Scale-

"There are some sentences related to your social and behavioral problems. These sentences are related to your day to day problems and experience. These sentences are not related to your intelligence test but to the test of some facts. Read carefully every problem. In front of every sentences there are 2 options 'yes' and 'No'. Tick mark the appropriate option according to your situation and behavior. You are totally free to fill the list. Your answer will be kept confidential. It is compulsory to answer all the questions."

Instructions of P.G.I. Health Questionnaire-

"There are some questions related to physical and mental health. Read carefully and tick mark those sentences which are appropriate for you."

3.8.2 Phase-II

Intervention Model

The following Dance Movement Therapy Intervention Model was prepared and used by the researcher in Phase-II. The sessions were provided for four-weeks duration. In each week, various techniques explained below were used by the researcher.

Table 3.6: Dance Movement Therapy Intervention Model

Week	Time	Techniques Used
First week	45 minutes per day	1. Warm-up 2. Dance 3. Stretching
Second week	45 minutes per day	1. Warm-up 2. Jumping with Music 3. Stretching 4. Breathing Exercise 5. Group Technique
Third week	45 minutes per day	1. Warm-up 2. Dance on Melodic music 3. Dance in Circle 4. Movement with props 5. Breathing Exercise 6. Stretching 7. Mirroring
Fourth week	45 minutes per day	1. Warm-up 2. Dance on Fast music 3. Movements in circle 4. Movements with props 5. Breathing exercise 6. Stretching 7. Mirroring

Dance Movement Therapy Techniques

Some techniques used in the intervention model have been explained below.

Warm-up – Warm-up is important to increase the body's core temperature, it also increasing the body's muscle temperature. Increasing muscle temperature is helpful to make the muscles flexible, nimble and malleable. A productive warm up also has the effect of increasing both heart rate and respiratory rate. This increases blood flow, which in turn increases the delivery of oxygen and nutrients to the working muscles. All this helps to prepare the muscles, tendons and joints for more strenuous activity. It includes- Head up and down, shoulder movement (both sides), both hands movement (both sides), waist movement (clock wise and anti-clock wise), legs movement, toes movement, jogging, walking on place etc.

Dance -After warm-up, Bollywood- Freestyle dance was done. Here, participants copied the therapist's dance moves. Therapist was doing dance steps and all were coping her steps. This was very fantastic session. Dance moves includes legs-hands movement, waist movements, it includes whole body movements. Those movements were done on randomly selected Bollywood songs.

Stretching- Stretching is the process of physical health and fitness it includes set down specific parts of the body into a position that will lengthen, or elongate, the muscles and associated soft tissues. Through regular stretching practice a number of changes start to occur within the body and specifically within the muscles themselves. Other tissues that start to adapt to the stretching process include the fascia, tendons, ligaments, skin and scar tissue.

Breathing exercise- In this exercise therapist practiced inhalation and escalation of breath. The therapist's instructions were "Let your Breath flow as deep down into your belly, without forcing it. Try breathing in through your nose and breathing out through mouth. Breathe in gently and regularly. Let it flow out gently."

Jumping with Music- Jumping is such a great exercise to reduce stress. Here, in the session Therapist made them jump in different sides like front jump, back jump, side jump on different tracks of music. The all participants were enjoying this jumping technique.

Group Technique-Group technique is where all members of session move in group. Therapist gave instructions to make a big circle and doing movements in circle as therapist was doing.

They all were moving in circle dancing in circle, doing different movements as therapist was doing. This group technique is useful to promote social well-being. It is beneficial to enhance social ability, cooperation, helping others, coordinate with others and ability to understand other's emotions.

Movement with props- In this technique therapist used different props like colorful ribbons and 'dupatta' in dance. Therapist and participants all were dancing on song with those props. These props lead happiness in participants. All participants were feeling joy and excitement by using those props. This joy and happiness are good for their mental health.

Mirroring- This technique is good to enhance emotional understanding and empathy for others. It this technique therapist imitate the movements of clients, their emotion and their intentions. This technique is commonly practiced in order to enhance empathy of the therapist for the client.

Instructions during DMT Intervention

The movements of this session were followed by some instructions. There were some instructions given by Therapist during session. These instructions were changed according to the sessions. These instructions were given when jumping and breathing exercises were conducted with movements:

"Bend your knees so they are released. Focus on your breath, notice how your body moves with your breath, move slowly, this is your body, you exist, find joy in bounce, bounce, bounce, you can play. When was the last time you jumped? Moves like nobody watching you, you are free totally free, move your spine, feel your spine, feel your heartbeat, its faster, you are alive, breathe, breathe deep breath, release your shoulder, find your inner rhythm, follow me, feel the movements, be brave, it doesn't matter how it all looks, take risks, just follow me. Refresh, follow me, feel your every movement, what are you holding in your hands, bring your negative world, can you compress them, can you crush them, I am crushing my negative vibes, this is my way, now they are dust, they are only thoughts, see how it feels to move this way on all the dust of negative words, I am crushing my negative words with my feet, give love to your body, you have healing power, breathe deep breathe, everything is alright, now we are focusing on our positive world, be focused on your positive thoughts, move with me, just follow me, draw the line of positivity, remember all positive words your positive thoughts, you are happy, you are very happy, you can tolerate everything, you can face everything, be prepare for every situation, just follow me, follow my moves, remember all love you gave your body, you are line, you are love, you are enough, you are a tree that can dance, that can move, move move, refresh, water heals your touch heals, give love to yourself, to your body, move through each parts to see it is okay, how did it change with movement, how did it change with words and exercises, today you gave the time yourself, thanks yourself, love yourself, deep breath and sit on the floor close your eyes feel your breathe, feel your body's energy, calm down feel the peace and relax."

3.9 ETHICAL ISSUES

- Informed Consent and Voluntary Participation: The dance trainee and non-dance trainee were informed about the study. They all knew about objectives of the study.
- Proper Rapport was established before the data collection for both the phases of the research.
- It was ensured that the confidentiality of the given information would be maintained.
- The researcher herself handled the psychological care and support during the data collection.
- The control group in the phase-II was also provided the dance movement therapy after the post-testing was over to offer similarity of treatment/benefits to the adolescents who had not received the DMT intervention earlier.

3.10 ANALYSIS OF DATA

The total scores for every scale for each respondent were obtained for all 120 adolescents after the data was over. For scoring procedures, the test manual of each of the Big Five Personality Test, Sinha Anxiety Scale and PGI Health Questionnaire was followed. After that, the data was entered into Microsoft Excel data sheet. The data which was entered included the demographic profile information as well the total scoress for all 120 people. Mean, S.D. and ANOVA were used for analyzing the data obtained in Phase-I and paired sample t-test was used to compare the control and experimental group in Phase-II.

For analyzing the data, Statistical Package for Social Scientists (SPSS) was used. For comprehending and interpreting the data, following statistical techniques were used.

Mean and Standard Deviation

The mean and standard deviation for personality and its big five traits, anxiety and psycho-physical health were obtained for adolescents dance trainees & non dance trainees. Similarly, the mean and standard deviation for personality, anxiety and psycho-physical health were obtained for male and female adolescents. For the ease of reading and understanding, Mean and S.D. were also presented graphically.

Analysis of Variance (ANOVA)

Analysis of Variance (ANOVA) is a compilation of statistical models and their correlated estimation procedures (like the "variation" among and between groups) used to figure out the differences among group means in a sample. ANOVA is useful in examining the main as well as the interaction of variables. Researchers have selected two independent variables, Gender and Dance Trainee, in the present research. ANOVA has enabled the research in studying the individual effects of each of the independent variables as well as the interaction effect of Gender and Dance Trainee on various dependent variables. A 2 x 2 factorial design has been used in this research to select samples; a two-way factorial ANOVA is appropriate for such types of designs. The p-value was calculated for the three dependent variables and was used for interpreting the level of significance for main as well as interactions effects.

t-test

To compare the mean of two groups, a statistical test called t-test is used. This test is generally used in hypothesis testing to know whether a treatment or process has an effect on the population of interest or whether one group is different from another. t-test is only used to compare the mean of 2 groups. Here, a paired sample t-test was used to as the same groups were pre and post tested on the variables.

CHAPTER 4

RESULT AND DISCUSSION

Result and Discussion section of any research is considered to be the most interesting yet a challenging task for the researcher. During this stage, all the efforts of the researcher; starting from selecting a relevant topic and determining research objectives till the scoring and analysis of the data; come to fruition. The researcher is also keen in finding out what are the main findings of the research.

Results section is focused on the main findings or direct answers to the research questions, mainly consisting of the statistical components. The detailed presentation of results in the form of tables and graphs leads to a better reader friendly presentation. Discussion completes the incomplete by explaining and interpreting the obtained findings, it finds out the meaning of the obtained results, why these results might have occurred, what are the contextual factors responsible, what are its supportive and contradictory findings etc.

A researcher can adopt various approaches while writing this chapter. Simultaneously presenting results and then explaining and discussing these results then and there so that it provides an opportunity to better relate and understand the findings. In this chapter, first results are presented in the form of tables and graphs which are followed by the discussion of the findings. In the discussion, the researcher puts own thought in making the findings more comprehensive. Discussion is looking at the results from more analytical, critical and interpretative perspective so that the final conclusions can be extracted from the research output. Conclusions are further the summary of the discussion which tells us what we learnt from the research. Drawing conclusions is more about winding up and giving a final touch to the obtained knowledge through the process of analysis, interpretation, synthesis, and evaluation. The conclusions of the present research work will be presented in the form of main findings separately in Chapter-6 : Summary.

4.1 OVERVIEW OF THE RESEARCH

This research has been conducted in two phases. In the first phases, 120 persons in the age group 18-30 years (with the mean age approximate 22 years) consisting of 60 dancers and 60 non-dancers were selected and were termed Dance Trainee (DT) and Non-dance Trainee (NDT) group. In each of the two groups, 30 male and 30 female were selected as per the 2 x 2 factorial designs. All the persons were administered with the selected tools to measure their Personality, Psychophysical health and the level of Anxiety.

In the second phase, 20 persons were selected from the NDT group and were randomly assigned to two groups; each group included 10 persons. It was also randomly decided which group would receive the treatment; hence control group and experimental group were also randomly decided. The experimental group was provided the Dance Movement Therapy (DMT) on the basis of Intervention Model prepared by the researcher. The effect of DMT intervention was studied on the Personality, Psychophysical health and the level of Anxiety.

4.2 FINDINGS OF THE STUDY

The findings of the present research were obtained by using various statistical techniques discussed in chapter-3. The findings are presented separately for both the phases of the research; Phase-I and Phase-II.

Phase-I

In this phase, the obtained results on the following variables from 120 persons have been discussed variable-wise.

1. Personality
2. Anxiety
3. Psychophysical health

4.2.1 Personality:

4.2.1.1 Frequency Distribution: NEO-Five Factors

Table 4.1: Different levels of Personality factors (NEO-FFI)

Level of Personality	Neuroticism	Extraversion	Openness	Agreeableness	Conscientiousness
Very high	Above 29	Above 36	Above 36	Above 40	Above 43
High	22-29	31-36	31-36	36-40	38-42
Average	13-21	24-30	23-30	29-35	30-37
Low	6-12	18-23	18-22	24-28	25-29
Very low	1-5	1-17	1-17	1-23	1-24

Table 4.2: Frequency Distribution of Five Factors of Personality (N=120)

Level of Personality	Number of respondents in different categories									
	N	%	E	%	O	%	A	%	C	%
Very high	54	45	29	24.16	3	2.5	0	0	0	0
High	33	27.5	17	14.16	11	9.16	21	17.5	6	5
Normal	32	26.6	47	39.16	41	34.16	18	15	36	30
Low	1	0.83	10	8.33	41	34.16	52	43.33	15	12.5
Very Low	0	0	17	14.16	24	20	29	24.16	63	52.5

N* Neuroticism, E*Extraversion, O*Openness, A*Agreeableness, C*Conscientiousness

The table 4.2 presents the number of persons falling in five categories from very high to very low for the total sample of 120 respondents. Some of the main observations from the data are as follows.

It is observed that 72.5% of the respondents are falling in either very high or high category on the level of neuroticism whereas only 26.6% respondents are falling in the normal category on Neuroticism. It shows that almost three fourth of the respondents exhibit high or very high neuroticism. High level of neuroticism is related with signs such as emotional reactivity, the tendency to get easily upset and irritated.

Such people are more prone to irrational ideas, and are less able to control their impulses and cope more poorly than others with stressful situations. These people also exhibit sub-traits such as anger, anxiety, self consciousness and vulnerability.

Among the total respondents, 77% have very high to high to normal levels of extraversion. These people enjoy working with people, are more outgoing. The respondents who are average on Extraversion, they are moderate in activity and enthusiasm. They enjoy the company of others but they also value privacy. Remaining 23% respondents have very low to low levels of extraversion. Such people are quiet and do not need any external stimulation to seek energy.

65% of the respondents have scored either very low or low on the Openness to Experience dimension of Big-five personality traits. Open to Experience includes active imagination, preference for variety of things and the readiness for intellectual curiosity and to prefer new experience than routine or familiar way of doing things. It means that 65% of the respondents have not shown these qualities. Only 11% of the respondents are high on Openness. 34% have scored average on this dimension. The persons who are average on Openness have quality of balancing between the old and the new. They are practical but willing to consider new ways of doing things.

From the total sample, 67.49% of respondents are low on Agreeableness. Low agreeableness is related with lack of the traits such as being cooperative and empathetic. Such people are more stubborn, skeptical, proud and competitive than others.

On the level of Conscientiousness, 65% of the respondents have scored very low to low. It shows that such people lack self discipline when it comes to planning and organizing their work. They also show traits such as irresponsibility and are not very well organized. Only 5% have shown high conscientiousness which is associated with the traits such as working diligently for the goals.

Tables 4.3 and 4.4 have presented the frequency distribution for five factors of personality for Non-dance trainees and Dance trainees groups as well.

Table 4.3: Five Factors of Personality for Non-Dance Trainees

(N=60)

Level of Personality	Number of Males (30)										Number of Females (30)									
	N	%	E	%	O	%	A	%	C	%	N	%	E	%	O	%	A	%	C	%
Very High	13	43.3	3	10	1	3.3	0	0	0	0	10	33.3	5	16.6	0	0	0	0	0	
High	7	23.3	3	10	3	10	2	6.6	2	6.66	13	43.3	5	16.6	5	16.6	7	23.3	3	10
Normal	10	33.3	11	36.6	10	33.3	5	16.5	10	33.3	7	23.3	15	50	10	33.3	6	20	8	26.6
Low	0	0	5	16.6	9	30	13	43.3	4	13.3	0	0	1	3.33	9	30	12	40	5	16.6
Very Low	0	0	8	26.6	7	23.3	10	33.3	14	46.6	0	0	4	13.3	6	20	5	16.6	14	46.6

N* Neuroticism, E*Extraversion, O*Openness, A*Agreeableness, C*Conscientiousness

The table 4.3 shows that from 30 male non dance trainees have 43.3% very high neuroticism level it means they are less able to control their impulses and they are very poor to cope up with their stress. They are more emotionally unstable in compare to those who got fewer score on Neuroticism. The table shows that from 30 male non dance trainees 20% respondents are very high on extraversion, 36.6% are having normal, 16.6% have low and 26.6% are having very low on extraversion level.

Some as, from 30 non male dance trainees 3.3% have very high openness level, 10% are high on openness level, 33.3% are having normal, 30% have low and 23.3% are very low on openness level. From some male categories 6.6% are high on Agreeableness, 16.5% are normal, 43.3% are low and 33.3% are very low on Agreeableness. Further, 6.66% are high on conscientiousness, 33.3% are normal, 13.3% are low and 46.6% are very low on conscientiousness. The table is also showing percentage level of female non-dance trainees (30). They are, from 30 non female dance trainees 33.3% are very high on neuroticism, 43.3% are high, 23.3% are normal on Neuroticism. Again from 30 non-dance female trainees 16.6% are very high on Extraversion, 16.6% are high, 50% are normal, 3.33% are low and 13.3% are very low on Extraversion. Some from these female non-dance trainees 16.6% are high on openness, 33.3% are normal, 30% are low and 20% are very low on openness. 23.3% are high on agreeableness, 20% are normal, 40% are low and 16.6% are very low on agreeableness. Among some females 10% are high on conscientiousness, 26.6% are normal, 16.6% are low and 46.6% are very low on conscientiousness.

Table 4.4: Five Factors of Personality for Dance Trainees (N=60)

Level of Personality	Number of Males (30)										Number of Females (30)									
	N	%	E	%	O	%	A	%	C	%	N	%	E	%	O	%	A	%	C	%
Very High	23	76.6	14	46.6	2	6.66	0	0	0	0	8	26.66	7	23.33	0	0	0	0	0	0
High	2	6.66	4	13.3	3	10	4	13.3	0	0	11	36.66	5	26.66	0	0	8	26.6	1	3.33
Normal	5	16.6	8	26.6	9	30	4	13.3	10	33.3	10	33.33	13	43.33	12	40	3	10	8	26.66
Low	0	0	1	3.33	12	40	16	53.3	4	13.33	1	3.33	3	10	11	36.6	11	36.6	2	6.66
Very Low	0	0	3	10	4	13.33	6	20	16	53.33	0	0	2	6.66	7	23.3	8	26.6	19	63.33

N* Neuroticism, E*Extraversion, O*Openness, A*Agreeableness, C*Conscientiousness

The table 4.4 shows that from 30 male dance trainees 76.6% have very high Neuroticism. 46.6% male Dance Trainee respondents are very high on Extraversion. They are more extraverted, outgoing, active and high-spirited respondents.

Further, from 30 female dance trainees only 26.66% are very high on Neuroticism, 36.66% are high, 33.33% are normal and 3.33% are low. Here we can say, from 30 male dance trainees 76.6% are very high on Neuroticism but from 30 female dance trainees there are only 26.66% are very high on Neuroticism. From the same 30 female dance trainees 23.33% are very high on Extraversion, 26.66% are high, 43.33% are normal, 10% are low and 6.66% are very low. 40% are normal on openness, 36.6% are low and 23.3% are very low. Further, from the same female group 26.6% are high on Agreeableness, 10% are normal, 36.6% are low and 26.6% are very low. For conscientiousness, 3.33% females are having high conscientiousness level, 26.66% are normal, 6.66% are low and 63.33% are very low.

4.2.1.2 Mean and Standard Deviation: Personality

The mean, standard deviations and Analysis of Variance for the following five factors of personality have been presented and discussed separately.

- Neuroticism
- Extraversion
- Agreeableness
- Openness
- Conscientiousness

Neuroticism

- As discussed in the previous section based on the frequency distribution, most of the respondents among total sample are Neurotic. They often feel helpless and want someone else to solve their problems. When things go wrong, they get discouraged and feel like giving up. However, it is important to understand the group differences on the level of neuroticism. The table 4.5 shows that the mean Neuroticism score of Dance Trainee female respondents is less than the mean Neuroticism of Non-Dance Trainee male respondents.

- The mean of Dance Trainee male respondents is higher than the mean of Non-Dance Trainee male respondents. It is surprising to note that the non-dancers have less neuroticism than dancers. Although this is due to the highest mean obtained for male dancers group which is 34.2 in comparison to 26.4 for male non-dancers. Among the four groups, male dancers have shown highest level of neuroticism.
- On the other hand, Female dancers have low neuroticism than female non-dancers; it shows that for female, dance training is helpful for low neuroticism.
- Male respondents are more neurotic than female respondents. The mean of Dance Trainee male respondents is higher than the mean of Dance Trainee female respondents. Female respondents are more emotionally stable than male respondents.

Table 4.5: Personality (Neuroticism) - Mean and SD

Gender	Trainee	Mean	Standard Deviation	N
Male	Non- Dance	26.46	7.28	30
	Dance	34.2	8.69	30
	Total	**30.33**	**8.85**	**60**
Female	Non- Dance	26.36	8.06	30
	Dance	23.53	8.64	30
	Total	**24.95**	**8.41**	**60**
Total	**Non- Dance**	**26.41**	**7.61**	**60**
	Dance	**28.86**	**10.14**	**60**
	Total	**27.64**	**8.60**	**120**

Graph 4.1 : Personality (Neuroticism) - Mean

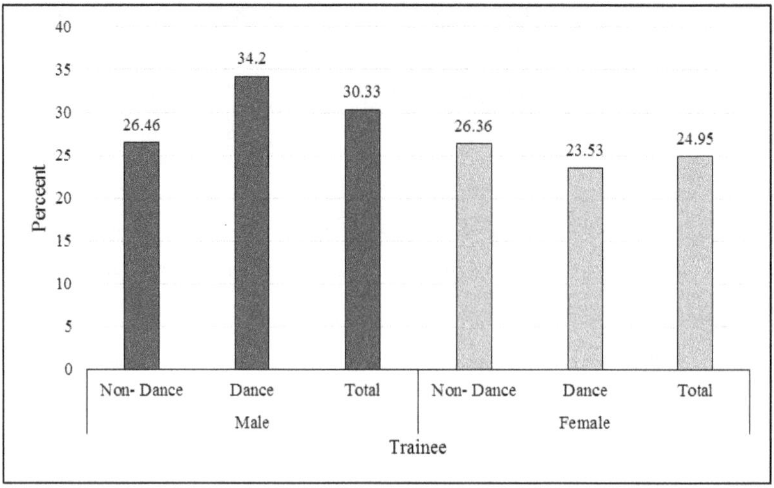

Analysis of Variance: Personality (Neuroticism)

The main aim of Analysis of Variance is to understand whether the means of different groups are statistically significant or not. In this research, a 2x2 factorial design has been used which permits for using a two-way factorial analysis of variance. The two independent variables are Dance Training (Dance Training and Non-Dance Training) and Gender (Male and Female).

The main effect of gender on Neuroticism was found significant at .01 levels. There was a significant effect of Gender on Neuroticism at $F=12.95$, $p<0.01$, there was significantly higher mean score of male (Mean=30.33, sd=8.858) than the mean score of female (mean=24.95, sd=8.412) on Neuroticism. It shows adolescents male have more negative feelings like fear, sadness, embarrassment, guilt, anger etc. in compared to female adolescents.

The main effect of dance training on Neuroticism was not found significant at .01 levels. There is no significantly effect of Dance Training on Neuroticism.

The interaction effect of gender and dance training on the level of neuroticism has been found significant at .01 levels. There was a significant effect of Gender and Dance Training on Neuroticism at $F=12.47$, $p<0.01$.

Table 4.6 - Personality (Neuroticism): Analysis of Variance

ANOVA						
Source of Variation	*Sum of Square*	*df*	*Mean Square*	*F*	*P-value*	*F crit*
Gender (Male & Female)	869.40	1	869.40	12.95	0.00	3.92
Dance Training (Dance trainee & Non-Dance Trainee)	180.07	1	180.07	2.68	0.10	3.92
Interaction effect (Gender * Dance Training	837.40	1	837.40	12.47	0.00	3.90
Within Groups	7786.7	116	67.12			
Total	**9673.59**	**119**				

Extraversion

- The table 4.7 shows that the mean Extraversion of dance trainee male is more than the mean of non-dance trainee male. The male respondents, who were going for any dance training, were more extravert than the male respondents who were not going for any dance training.
- The mean score of Dance Trainee female respondents is more than the mean score of non-dance trainee female respondents.
- For both the male and female respondents, dance Trainee respondents are more extravert in their behavior in comparison to their respective counterparts.
- On the basis of gender, the mean scores of extraversion are 28.16 and 28.7 respectively for male and female respondents. It shows that these groups do not differ on the level of extraversion. It would further be discussed with ANOVA results.
- Among the four groups, the male dancers group has shown higher level of extraversion whereas the male non-dancers group has shown lowest level of extraversion. The mean of Dance Trainee male respondents is more than the mean of Dance Trainee female respondents. It shows the male Dance Trainee respondents are more extravert than the female dance trainee respondents.

Table 4.7: Personality (Extraversion) - Mean and SD

Gender	Trainee	Mean	Standard Deviation	N
Male	Non- Dance	24.16	8.16	30
	Dance	32.16	9.22	30
	Total	28.16	9.47	60
Female	Non- Dance	28.06	7.88	30
	Dance	29.33	7.88	30
	Total	28.7	7.63	60
Total	**Non- Dance**	**26.11**	**8.13**	**60**
	Dance	**30.75**	**8.49**	**60**
	Total	**20.27**	**8.60**	**120**

Graph 4.2: Personality (Extraversion) - Mean

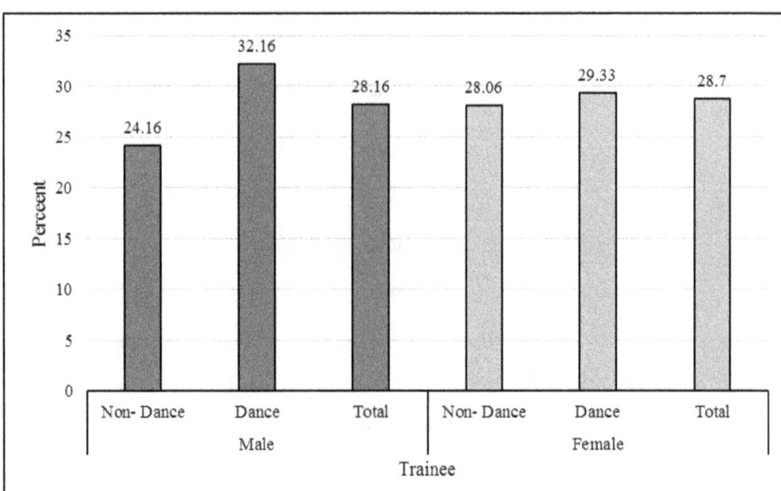

Table 4.8 Personality (Extraversion): Analysis of Variance

ANOVA						
Source of Variation	*Sum of Square*	*df*	*Mean Square*	*F*	*P-value*	*F crit*
Gender (Male & Female)	8.53	1	8.53	0.12	0.72	3.92
Dance Training (Dance trainee & Non-Dance Trainee)	644.03	1	644.03	9.55	0.00	3.92
Interaction effect (Gender * Dance Training)	340.03	1	340.03	5.04	0.02	3.92
Within Groups	7816.86	116	67.38			
Total	**8809.46**	**119**				

The main effect of Dance Training on Extraversion was found significant at 0.01 levels. The dance trainees exhibited more Extraversion than the non-dance trainees. There was a significant effect of Dance Training on Extraversion at $F=9.55$, $p<0.01$, there was significantly higher mean score of Extraversions on dance trainee respondents ($M=30.75$, S.D. = 8.49) than the mean score of Non-Dance Trainee. ($M=26.12$, S.D. = 8.13). Dance Training has significantly affected extraversion. Dancing is a great path to make new friends. It is good social environment where one can easily express his feelings.

The main effect of gender on Extraversion was not found significant.

The interaction effect of Gender and Dance Training on Extraversion was found significant at 0.05 levels There was a significant interaction effect of Gender and Dance Training on Extraversion at $F=5.04$, $p<0.05$. It shows that gender is interacting with dance training to influence extraversion. When the male respondents involve in dance training, their extraversion levels would be higher in comparison to female involved in dance training.

Openness to Experience

- The table 4.9 shows that the Mean Openness score of various groups do not differ much and are close to the overall group (N=120) mean 22.32.
- Table 4.10 shows that the main effect of Dance Training on Openness was not found significant. There is no effect of Dance Training on Openness. Similarly, the main effect of Gender on Openness was also not found significant. There is no effect of gender on Openness. The interaction effect of gender and dance training on openness is also not found significant.

Table 4.9: Personality (Openness) - Mean and SD

Gender	Trainee	Mean	Standard Deviation	N
Male	Non- Dance	22.9	6.25	30
	Dance	22.83	5.97	30
	Total	**22.86**	**6.06**	**60**
Female	Non- Dance	23.43	6.40	30
	Dance	20.13	3.69	30
	Total	**21.78**	**5.44**	**60**
Total	**Non- Dance**	**23.16**	**6.28**	**60**
	Dance	**21.48**	**5.10**	**60**
	Total	**22.32**	**5.76**	**120**

Graph 4.3: Personality (Openness) - Mean

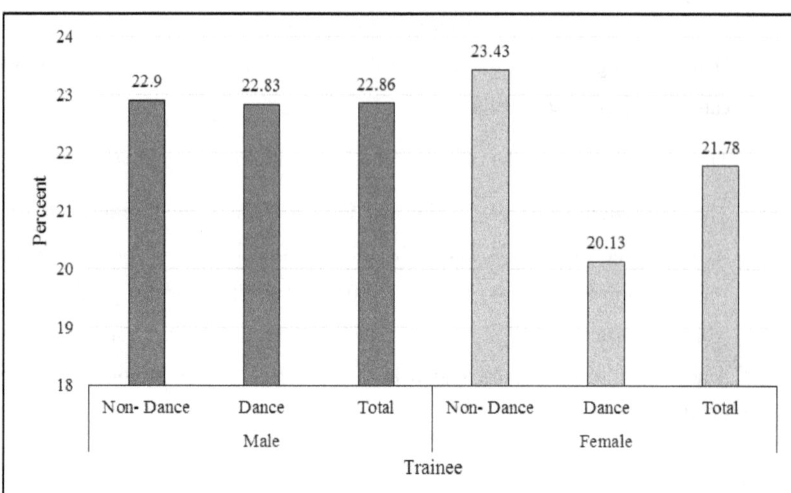

Table 4.10 Personality (Openness): Analysis of Variance

ANOVA						
Source of Variation	***Sum of Square***	***df***	***Mean Square***	***F***	***P-value***	***F crit***
Gender (Male & Female)	35.20	1	35.20	1.08	0.29	3.92
Dance Training (Dance trainee & Non-Dance Trainee)	85.00	1	85.00	2.62	0.10	3.92
Interaction effect (Gender * Dance Training	78.40	1	78.40	2.42	0.12	3.92
Within Groups	3755.7	116	32.37			
Total	**3954.32**	**119**				

Agreeableness

- The table 4.11 shows that the Mean Agreeableness score of various groups do not differ much and are close to the overall group (N=120) mean 26.35.
- Table 4.12 shows that the main effect of Dance Training on Agreeableness was not found significant. There is no effect of Dance Training on Agreeableness. Similarly, the main effect of Gender on Agreeableness was also not found significant. There is no effect of gender on Agreeableness. The interaction effect of gender and dance training on Agreeableness is also not found significant.

Table 4.11: Personality (Agreeableness) - Mean and SD

Gender	Trainee	Mean	Standard deviation	N
Male	Non- Dance	24.7	5.34	30
	Dance	25.8	6.80	30
	Total	25.25	6.11	60
Female	Non- Dance	28.16	6.99	30
	Dance	26.73	6.99	30
	Total	27.45	7.62	60
Total	**Non- Dance**	**26.43**	**6.41**	**60**
	Dance	**26.26**	**7.53**	**60**
	Total	**26.35**	**6.96**	**120**

Graph 4.4: Personality (Agreeableness) - Mean

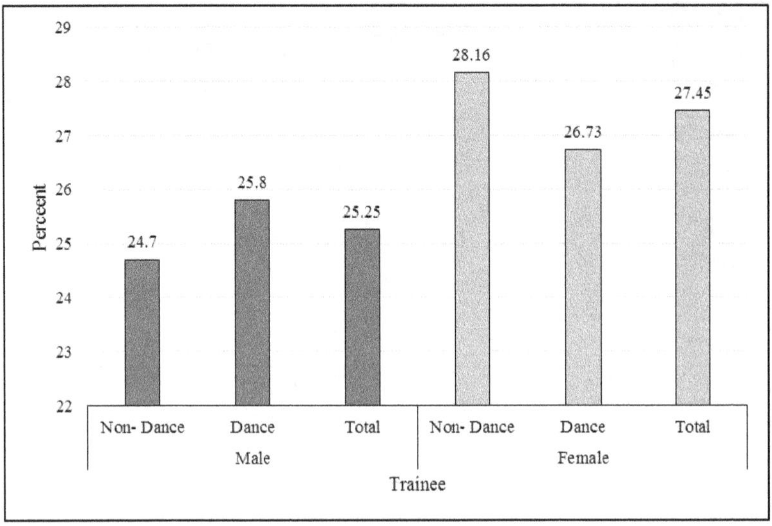

Table 4.12 Personality (Agreeableness): Analysis of Variance

ANOVA						
Source of Variation	*Sum of Square*	*df*	*Mean Square*	*F*	*P-value*	*F crit*
Gender (Male & Female)	145.2	1	145.2	3.01	0.08	3.92
Dance Training (Dance trainee & Non-Dance Trainee)	0.83	1	0.83	0.01	0.89	3.92
Interaction effect (Gender * Dance Training	48.13	1	48.13	0.99	0.31	3.92
Within Groups	5585.13	116	48.14			
Total	**5779.3**	**119**				

Conscientiousness

- The table 4.13 shows that the Mean Agreeableness score of various groups do not differ much and are close to the overall group (N=120) mean 26.63.
- Table 4.14 shows that the main effect of Dance Training on Conscientiousness was not found significant. There is no effect of Dance Training on Conscientiousness. Similarly, the main effect of Gender on Conscientiousness was also not found significant. There is no effect of gender on Conscientiousness. The interaction effect of gender and dance training on Conscientiousness is also not found significant.

Table 4.13: Personality (Conscientiousness) - Mean and SD

Gender	Trainee	Mean	Standard Deviation	N
Male	Non- Dance	26.76	7.16	30
	Dance	27	6.00	30
	Total	26.88	6.55	60
Female	Non- Dance	26.96	6.77	30
	Dance	25.8	7.5	30
	Total	26.38	7.12	60
Total	**Non- Dance**	**26.86**	**6.91**	**60**
	Dance	**26.4**	**6.77**	**60**
	Total	**26.63**	**6.82**	**120**

Graph 4.5: Personality (Conscientiousness) - Mean

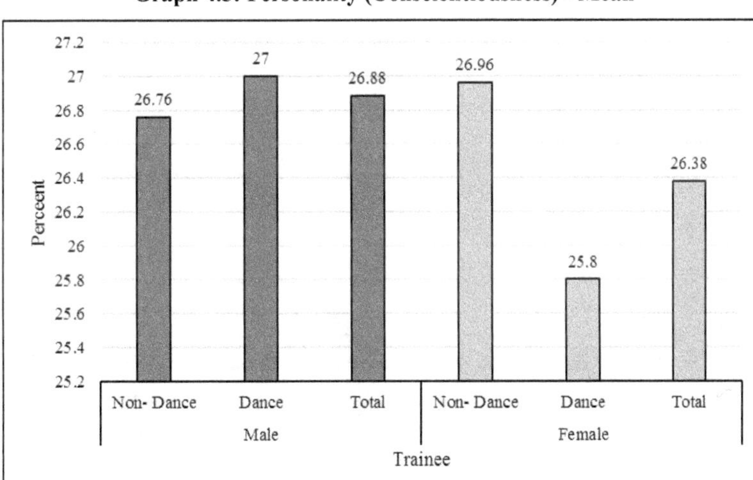

Table 4.14 Personality (Conscientiousness): Analysis of Variance

ANOVA						
Source of Variation	*Sum of Square*	*df*	*Mean Square*	*F*	*P-value*	*F crit*
Gender (Male & Female)	7.5	1	7.5	0.15	0.69	3.92
Dance Training (Dance trainee & Non-Dance Trainee)	6.53	1	6.53	0.13	0.71	3.92
Interaction effect (Gender * Dance Training	14.7	1	14.7	0.30	0.57	3.92
Within Groups	5507.13	116	47.47			
Total	**5535.66**	**119**				

4.2.2 Anxiety

4.2.2.1 Frequency Distribution

Table 4.15: Level of anxiety for the total sample (N=120)

Level of Anxiety	**Number of respondents (N=120)**	**Percentage**
Very high	0	0
High	11	9.16
Normal	56	46.66
Low	34	28.33
Very low	19	15.83

The table 4.12 shows that 46.66% have normal anxiety, 28.33% low anxiety, 15.83 % very low anxiety and 9.16% are having very high anxiety level.

Table 4.16: Levels of Anxiety for the Non-Dance Trainee Group (N=60)

Level of Anxiety	Number of males (N=30)	Percentage	Number of females (N=30)	Percentage	Total respondents (n=60)	Percentage
Very high	0	0	0	0	0	0
High	5	16.66	6	20	11	18.33
Normal	12	40	12	40	24	40
Low	10	33.33	9	30	19	31.66
Very low	3	10	3	10	6	10

Table 4.17: Levels of Anxiety for the Dance Trainees Group (N=60)

Level of Anxiety	Number of males (N=30)	Percentage (%)	Number of females (N=30)	Percentage	Total respondents (n=60)	Percentage (%)
Very high	0	0	0	0	0	0
High	0	0	0	0	0	0
Normal	18	60	14	46.66	32	53.33
Low	6	20	9	30	15	25
Very low	6	20	7	23.33	13	21.66

4.2.2.3 Mean and Standard Deviation: Anxiety

- The table 4.18 shows the mean Anxiety score of Dance Trainee group is less than the mean of Non-Dance Trainee group. It shows Dance Training group has less anxiety.
- The Dance Trainee respondents are more optimistic than Non-Dance Trainee respondents. They can sleep easily without any tension. They are mentally stronger than Non-Dance Trainee respondents. They never worried about small things. They believe in positivity more than Non-Dance Trainee respondents.
- The female respondents have more Anxiety than male respondents, however, this difference is not found to be statistically significant.

Table 4.18: Mean and Standard Deviation - Anxiety

Gender	Trainee	Mean	Standard Deviation	N
Male	Non- Dance	25.7	7.40	30
	Dance	22.73	5.80	30
	Total	24.21	6.76	60
Female	Non- Dance	28.53	9.09	30
	Dance	22.5	4.89	30
	Total	25.51	7.85	60
Total	**Non- Dance**	**27.11**	**8.34**	**60**
	Dance	**22.61**	**5.32**	**60**
	Total	**20.27**	**8.08**	**120**

Table 4.6: Anxiety – Mean

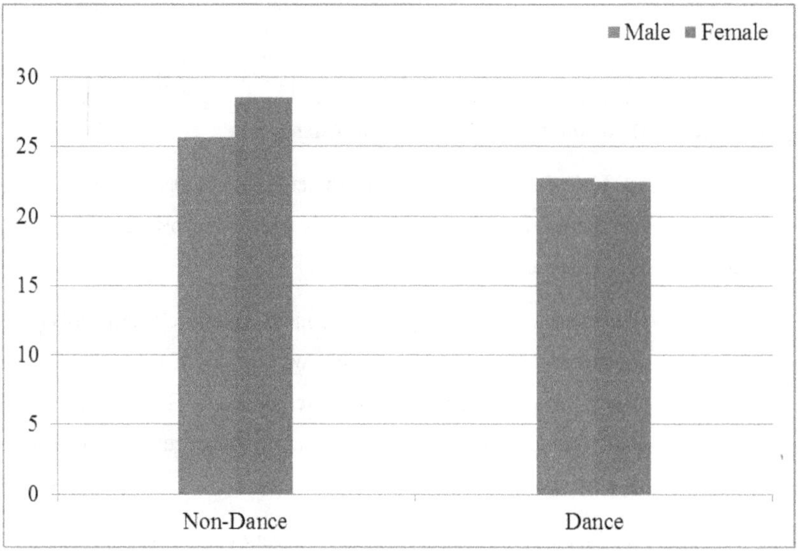

4.2.2.4 Analysis of Variance: Anxiety

Table 4.19 Analysis of Variance - Anxiety

ANOVA						
Source of Variation	*Sum of Square*	*df*	*Mean Square*	*F*	*P-value*	*F crit*
Gender (Male & Female)	50.7	1	50.7	1.0385	0.31029	3.922
Dance Training (Dance trainee & Non-Dance Trainee)	607.5	1	607.5	12.443	0.000602	3.922
Interaction effect (Gender * Dance Training	70.533	1	70.533	1.444	0.231819	3.922
Within Groups	5663.133	116	48.820			
Total	**6391.866**	**119**				

Dance Training and Anxiety

Table 4.20 shows that the main effect of dance training on anxiety was found significant at .01 levels. The respondents who were undergoing dance training, experienced less anxiety as compared to those who were not taking any dance training. There was a significant effect of dance training on anxiety at F= 12.44, p< .000, there was significantly higher mean score of anxiety on non-dance trainee respondents (M= 27.11, S.D. 8.34) than the mean score of dance trainee respondents (M= 22.61, S.D.= 5.32). The result concluded that dance training is good for decreasing anxiety level in respondents.

Gender and Anxiety:

The main effect of Gender on Anxiety was not found significant. There was non-significant effect of Gender on Anxiety at F=1.03, p=0.31.

Interaction Effect:

The interaction effect of gender and dance training on Anxiety was also not found to be significant. There is no difference in the level of Anxiety among male and female who were going for dance training. There was non-significant interaction effect of Gender and dance training on Anxiety at F=1.444, p=0.23.

4.2.3 Psychophysical Health

4.2.3.1 Mean and Standard Deviation: Psychophysical Health

Physical Health

- The table 4.21 shows mean Physical health of Dance Trainee respondents is less than the mean of Non-Dance Trainee respondents. The less the score is, the better the Physical health is.
- The Dance Trainee respondents have better physical health than the Non-Dance Trainee respondents. Dance is best exercise for our body. Respondents become more flexible and fit through Dance. Dance Training increased muscular strength, improve posture and flexibility. It is also helpful in reduce pain and stiffness.
- The female respondents have better Physical health than the male respondents.
- Male Dance Trainee respondents are more physically fit than female Dance Trainee respondents. Male Dance Trainee respondents feel less Dizziness than others. They are not much worried about their health. They are less suffering from headache and other physical health related problems than their comparison group.
- Among the four groups, male dance trainee groups showed best physical health whereas male non-dancers suffered the most with physical health related issues.

Table 4.20: Mean and Standard Deviation: Physical Health

Gender	Trainee	Mean	Standard Deviation	N
Male	Non- Dance	7.43	2.35	30
	Dance	0.86	0.93	30
	Total	4.15	3.75	60
Female	Non- Dance	5.33	1.34	30
	Dance	1.43	1.50	30
	Total	3.38	2.42	60
Total	**Non- Dance**	**6.38**	**2.17**	**60**
	Dance	**1.15**	**1.27**	**60**
	Total	**3.76**	**3.17**	**120**

Graph 4.7: Physical Health – Mean

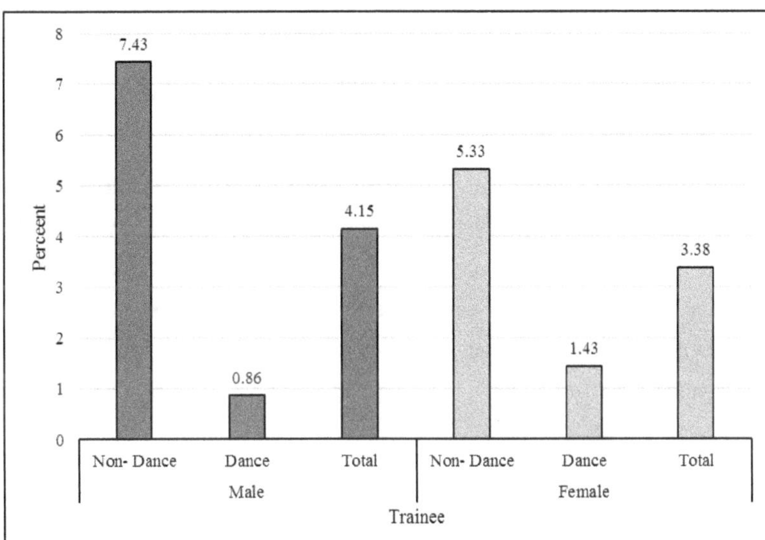

Table 4.21 Analysis of Variance: Physical Health

ANOVA						
Source of Variation	*Sum of Square*	*df*	*Mean Square*	*F*	*P-value*	*F crit*
Gender (Male & Female)	821.63	1	821.63	312.62	.000	3.92
Dance Training (Dance trainee & Non-Dance Trainee)	17.63	1	17.63	6.70	0.025	3.92
Interaction effect (Gender * Dance Training	53.33	1	53.33	20.29	.000	3.92
Within Groups	304.86	116	2.62			
Total	**1197.46**	**119**				

The main effect of Dance training on Physical health was found significant at 0.01 levels. There was a significant effect of Dance training on Physical health at F=6.70, p=0.01, there was significantly higher mean score of non-dance trainees (Mean=6.38, S.D. =2.17) than the mean score of dance trainees (mean=1.15, S.D.=1.27) on Physical health.

The main effect of Gender on Physical health was found significant at 0.01 levels. There was a significant effect of Gender on Physical health at F=312.62, p<0.00, there was significantly higher mean score of male respondents (Mean=4.15, S.D. =3.75) than the mean score of female (mean=3.35, S.D.=2.42) on Physical health. The interaction effect of Gender and Dance Training on Physical health was also found significant at 0.01 levels.

Mental Health

- The table 4.22 shows Dance Trainee respondents have good mental health than Non-Dance Trainee respondents. The Dance Trainee respondents can easily adjust in any situation than others. They are able to handle every situation with positivity. They have more control on their emotions in compare to Non-Dance Trainee respondents. Similarly, female respondents have better mental health the male respondents. Among the four groups, the male dance trainee groups showed the best mental health whereas the male non-dance trainee group suffered the most with mental health related issues.

- Table 4.23 shows that the main effect of Dance training on Mental health was found significant at 0.01 levels. There was a significant effect of Dance training on Mental health at F=338.77, $p<0.000$, there was significantly higher mean score of non-dance trainees (Mean=8.03, S.D. =3.61) than the mean score of dance trainees (mean=1.2, S.D.=1.05) on Mental health.
- Table 4.23 also shows that the main effect of Gender on Mental health was found significant at 0.01 levels. There was a significant effect of Gender on Mental health at F=6.70, $p<0.05$, there was significantly higher mean score of male respondents (Mean=5.78, S.D. =5.29) than the mean score of female (mean=3.45, S.D.=2.66) on Mental health. The interaction effect of Gender and Dance Training on Mental health was also found significant at 0.01 levels.

Table 4.22: Mean and Standard Deviation- Mental Health

Gender	Trainee	Mean	Standard Deviation	N
Male	Non- Dance	10.46	3.61	30
	Dance	1.1	0.84	30
	Total	5.78	5.29	60
Female	Non- Dance	5.6	1.83	30
	Dance	1.3	1.2	30
	Total	3.45	2.66	60
Total	**Non- Dance**	**8.03**	**3.61**	**60**
	Dance	**1.2**	**1.05**	**60**
	Total	**8.03**	**4.33**	**120**

Graph 4.8 : Mental Health – Mean

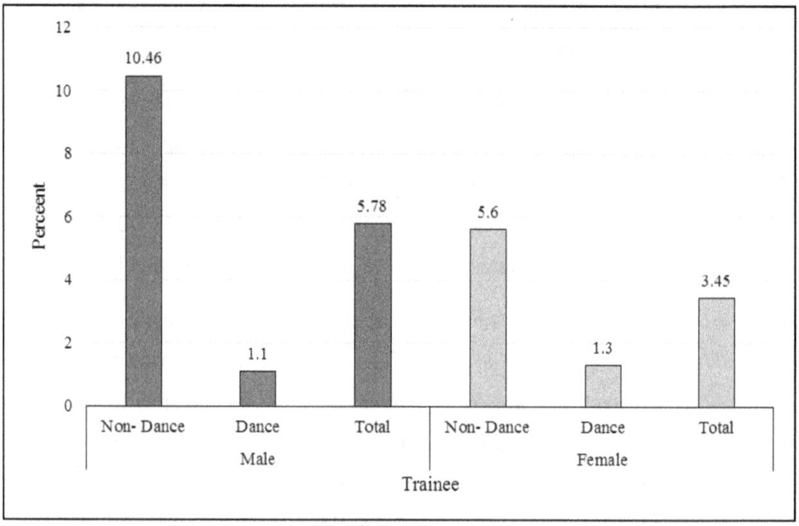

Table 4.23 Analysis of Variance - Mental Health

ANOVA						
Source of Variation	*Sum of Square*	*df*	*Mean Square*	*F*	*P-value*	*F crit*
Gender (Male & Female)	163.33	1	163.33	39.49	.000	3.92
Dance Training (Dance trainee & Non-Dance Trainee)	1400.83	1	1400.83	338.77	.000	3.92
Interaction effect (Gender * Dance Training	192.53	1	192.53	46.56	.000	3.92
Within Groups	479.66	116	4.13			
Total	**2236.36**	**119**				

Psychophysical Health

This section presents results for Psychophysical health which represents the overall health scores obtained from the total scores of Area A i.e. Physical health and Area B i.e. Mental Health.

Table 4.24: Mean and Standard deviation: Dance Training and Psychophysical Health

	N	Mean	Deviation	Std. Error	df	p. Value
Dance Trainee	60	2.35	2.073	0.268		
Non-Dance Trainee	60	14.40	5.228	0.675	118	0.000

Graph 4.9 : Dance Training and Psychophysical Health - Mean

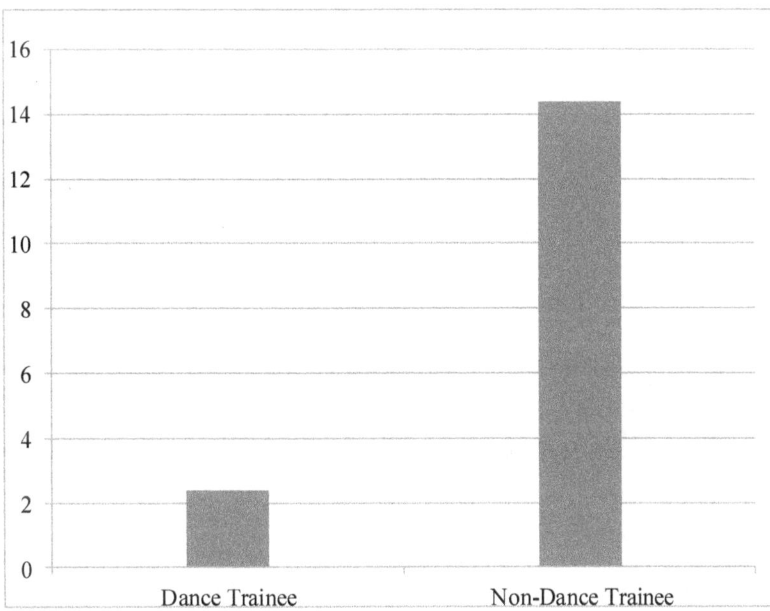

- Table 4.24 shows the Psychophysical Health of Dance Trainee respondents is better in comparison to the Non-Dance Trainee respondents.

Table 4.25: Mean and Standard Deviation: Gender and Psychophysical Health

	N	Mean	Deviation	Std. Error	df	p. Value
Male	60	10.30	8.504	1.098		
Female	60	6.45	5.060	0.653	118	0.003

Graph 4.10: Gender and Psychophysical Health - Mean

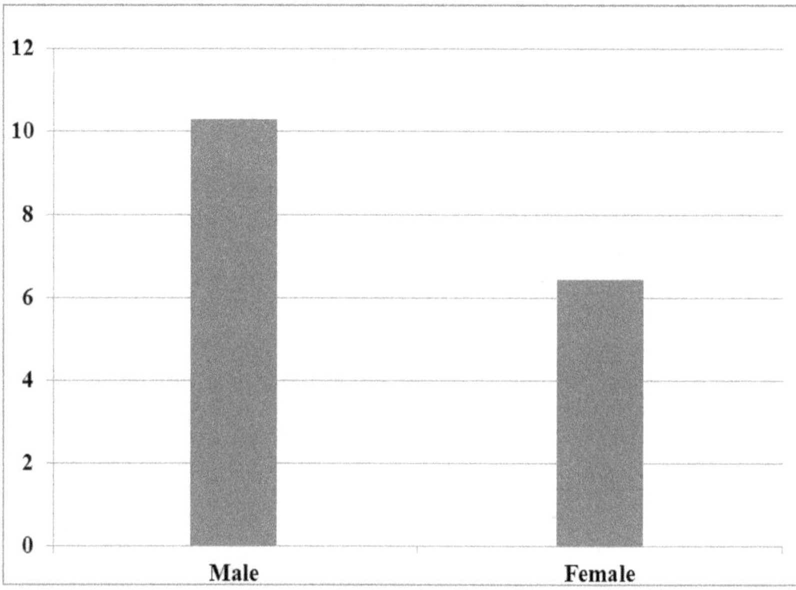

- The table 4.25 shows Gender and P.G.I. total Psychophysical health scores. The mean of male respondents is 10.30 and the mean of female respondents is 6.45. The mean of female is less than the mean of male respondents. The female respondents are more physically and mentally fit in comparison to male respondents.

4.2.3.2 Analysis of Variance: Psychophysical Health

The main effect of dance training of Psychophysical health was found significant at 0.01 levels. The respondents, who were going for dance training, were physically and mentally health as compared to those who were not taking any dance training. There was a significant effect of dance training on Psychophysical health at F=257.96, P<0.000, the result concluded that dance training is good for physical health of respondents. The respondents, who were going for dance training, were mentally health as compared to those who were not taking any dance training. Constant movements during dance results into improve cardiovascular functioning. During dance the heart beat as faster as, fast dance is done which makes heart strong and healthier. Lower body strength and overall core strength can be improving with the help of dance as it requires fancy footwork which is excellent for legs and core strength. Dance has positive impact on the mind too. Moving on favorite song, gives us happiness, and we are able to reconnect with over selves. The main effect of Gender on Psychophysical health was found significant at 0.05 levels. The result concluded that female respondents are more physically and mentally health in compared to male respondents. The interaction effect of Gender and Dance Training on Psychophysical Health was not found to be significant.

Phase-II

Intervention Phase: Dance Movement Therapy

In the second phase, 20 persons were selected from the Non-dance trainees' group and were randomly assigned to two groups; each group included 10 persons. It was also randomly decided which group would receive the treatment; hence control group and experimental group were also randomly decided.

Pre-testing data for all the three dependent variables was already available from Phase-I. Post-testing data was obtained after the intervention model implemented on the experimental group. The experimental group was provided dance-movement therapy sessions for four weeks by using the techniques mentioned in the proposed intervention model prepared by the researcher. The intervention model and its techniques have already been discussed in detail in Chapter-3. The effect of DMT intervention was studied on the Personality, Psychophysical health and the level of Anxiety. The significance of the difference between means of both control and experimental group was studied by using t-test. The results obtained for Phase-II will be discussed now.

Intervention Phase Results

(1) Personality

(a) Neuroticism

Table 4.26: Neuroticism and Dance Movement Therapy

Control Group		Experimental group	
Pretest score	Post test score	Pretest score	Post test score
Mean=23.4	Mean=23.2	Mean=19.9	Mean=17.9
0.79		0.02 Significant	

The effect of dance movement therapy on Neuroticism was found significant at 0.02 levels. There was a significant effect of dance movement therapy on Neuroticism in the experimental group. The difference in the neuroticism levels among the control group did not differ significantly. It can be concluded that the neuroticism level decreased in the experimental group due to the intervention in the form of dance movement therapy. The result shows dance movement Therapy effect Neuroticism. Neuroticism includes feeling of fear, jealousy, guilt, anger, worry, frustration and loneliness etc. It is possible to manage these negative feelings through dance movement therapy.

(b) Extraversion

Table 4.27: Extraversion and Dance Movement Therapy

Control Group		Experimental group	
Pretest score	Post test score	Pretest score	Post test score
Mean=28.9	Mean=26	Mean=24.9	Mean=30.4
0.37		0.00 Significant	

The effect of dance movement therapy on extraversion was found significant at 0.00 levels. There was a significant effect of dance movement therapy on Extraversion. The experimental group which had undergone dance movement therapy sessions reported high levels of extraversion. It indicates dance can help to increase the extraversion. It was seen that the experimental group who had been undergoing dance movement therapy for 3 months, they were easily able to talk to others, and they would quickly mix with others.

(c) Openness

Table 4.28: Openness and Dance Movement Therapy

Control Group		Experimental group	
Pretest score	Post test score	Pretest score	Post test score
Mean=24.1	Mean=24.1	Mean=23.5	Mean=23.5
		Non-significant	

The effect of dance movement therapy on openness was not found significant. There was non-significant effect of dance movement therapy on openness.

(d) Agreeableness

Table 4.29: Agreeableness and Dance Movement Therapy

Control Group		Experimental group	
Pretest score	Post test score	Pretest score	Post test score
Mean=27.8	Mean=27.8	Mean=26	Mean=24.6
		Non-significant	

The effect of dance movement therapy on Agreeableness was not found significant. The dance movement therapy has no effect on tendency of Agreeableness.

(e) Conscientiousness

Table 4.30: Conscientiousness and Dance Movement Therapy

Control Group		Experimental group	
Pretest score	Post test score	Pretest score	Post test score
Mean=28.2	Mean=27.2	Mean=26.6	Mean=26.1
		Non-significant	

The effect of dance movement therapy on conscientiousness was not found significant. The pre-test and post-test mean of experimental groups did not differ significantly.

(2) Anxiety

Table 4.31: Anxiety and Dance Movement Therapy

Control Group		Experimental group	
Pretest score	Post test score	Pretest score	Post test score
Mean=21.6	Mean=17.2	Mean=20.3	Mean=18.2
0.02 Significant		0.02 Significant	

Here, the level of anxiety in both groups is decreasing in post-test, it means the level of anxiety is decreasing but it cannot be concluded that the decrease in the level of anxiety is due to dance movement therapy intervention; because this decrease is also reported in the control group which is also significant.

(3) Psychophysical Health

Table 4.32: Physical Health and Dance Movement Therapy

Control Group		Experimental group	
Pretest score	Post test score	Pretest score	Post test score
Mean=4.4	Mean=3.4	Mean=5.9	Mean=3.9
0.12 Non-significant		0.00 Significant	

The effect of dance movement therapy on Physical Health was found significant at 0.00 levels. There was a significant effect of dance movement therapy on physical health. There was significantly lower mean score of experimental groups post-test (M=3.9) in comparison to the pre-test (M=5.9). Lower scores means better physical health. The mean value of control group (m=3.4) is also decreasing in post-test but this difference in the pre-test and post-test scores of the control group is not significant. It can be concluded that dance movement therapy is helpful in improving physical health. Movements are good for muscles strength, body flexibility and to reduce fat.

Table 4.33: Mental Health and Dance Movement Therapy

Control Group		Experimental group	
Pretest score	Post test score	Pretest score	Post test score
Mean=4.4	Mean=2.6	Mean=10.7	Mean=6.2
0.01 Significant		0.000 Significant	

The mean Mental health scores of both groups are decreasing that means the mental health has shown improvements in both control and experimental groups; hence it cannot be concluded that Dance Movement Therapy has resulted in improvement in mental health. Although the difference in the experimental group is statistically significant at .000 levels in comparison to the control group where the means values differ significantly at .01 levels. The means scores have improved from 10.7 to 6.2 in the experimental group in comparison to the control groups where the mean mental health score have improved from 4.4 to 2.6. It shows that DMT has posed better improvement in the mental health.

On the basis of the above results, the following observations can be drawn.

- Therapeutic Dance is good for decreasing Neuroticism level and increasing Extraversion in behaviour. The different techniques of session help to positively affect these dimensions of the participants' personality. They help to develop social skills as well as the ability to regulate one's emotional reactivity, impulsivity, anger etc.
- Therapeutic Dance is also good to remain physically healthy. Dance is a good exercise. Through dance exercise one can reduce fat and remain healthy and fit. Stretching is good to make body more flexible. Breathing exercise is beneficial to reduce stress. DMT has also found to be effective in improving mental health.

Participants' Experiences about DMT

When researcher asked the participants about their experiences of dancing regularly since last 4 weeks, they said they feel relaxed and they felt more connected to themselves and they didn't want to leave the dance class as long as possible. It gives them instant relief. The respondents who were in the job somewhere, they told the researcher that after office time, when they join dance class daily, they feel refresh, energetic and when they practice 'cool down' in dance session, they feel calm and relaxed. The researcher also talked to some choreographers, Rajasthan, they told that whenever they were anxious, they do practice Dance.

4.3 HYPOTHESIS TESTING:

This section represents Hypothesis testing, in which researcher found through obtained results, whether hypothesis have been accepted or rejected.

1. There is no difference between the personality of dance trainee and non-dance trainee.

➢ This null hypothesis has been partially accepted and partially rejected. The difference in extraversion is found to be significantly different between dance trainees and non-dance trainees; but the these groups do not differ significantly on the other four factors Neuroticism, Openness, Agreeableness and Conscientiousness.

2. There is no difference between the psychophysical health of dance training and non-dance training.

➢ This hypothesis has been rejected as the mean of dance trainee on psychophysical health is less than the mean of non-dance trainee. The effect of dance training on psychophysical health was found significant at 0.000 levels. There is difference between the psychophysical health of dance trainee and non-dance trainee, where the dance trainees have better psychophysical health than the non-dance trainee group.

3. There is no difference between the level of anxiety of dance trainee and non-dance trainee.

➢ This null hypothesis has been rejected as there is difference between the level of anxiety of dance trainee and non-dance trainee. the anxiety of non-dance trainee is more than the level of anxiety among dance trainees. The effect of dance training on Anxiety was found significant at 0.000 levels.

4. There is no difference between the personality of males and females.

➢ This null hypothesis has been partially accepted and partially rejected as there is no difference between the personality of males and females on four of the five factors i.e. extraversion, openness, agreeableness and conscientiousness; however the effect of Gender on Neuroticism was found significant at 0.001 levels.

5. There is no difference between the psychophysical health of males and females.

➢ This null hypothesis has been rejected as the Psychophysical health of female respondents is better than the male respondents. There is difference between the psychophysical health of males and females. The effect of gender on Psychophysical health was found significant at 0.01 levels.

6. There is no difference between the level of anxiety of males and females.

➢ This null hypothesis has been accepted as there is no difference between the level of anxiety of males and females. The effect of gender on anxiety was found non-significant.

7. There is no effect of therapeutic use of dance movement therapy on personality, psychophysical health and anxiety.

This hypothesis is partially accepted and partially rejected. The therapeutic use of dance movement therapy has significantly affected neuroticism and extraversion dimension among the five factors of personality. The other three factors openness, agreeableness and conscientiousness have not been affected significantly by the dance movement therapy intervention. The DMT intervention has also not affected the level of anxiety and mental health. However, the physical health as improved due to the intervention.

4.4 FURTHER DISCUSSION

Dance is a form of physical exercise. An individual involves not only physically in the dancing but the other aspects such as mental, cognitive and affective domains are also involved. This further strengthens an individual's psychomotor aspects. It provides body balance and coordination to the body. When a dancer remembers certain steps and techniques of dancing, it strengthens various cognitive activities such as attention, concentration, memory, thinking etc.

As a form of physical activity, many dance classes organize dance sessions for various other dance forms. It provides flexibility to the body, it leads to better blood circulation, sweating and cleansing of the body fluids. It revitalizes and rejuvenates the body. Cardiovascular benefits of physical exercises are also obtained in the process of dancing. Dance exercise is helpful in strengthening our bones and muscles. Increased level of physical activity can help intercept illness such as diabetes, heart disease and reduce the risk of osteoporosis as bones become stronger. These reasons lead to improvement in the Physical health due to dance.

When an individual engages in dance practice, it poses challenges to the individual's brain. Focusing on certain steps and being able to follow those steps and techniques requires body coordination and cognitions. Recalling the constant changing movement in the desired sequence requires the brain to function faster. The brain works on both sensory and motor functions, cognitive functions which improves the neural circuits in the brain. Dance is, thus the best form of mental exercise also. A study published in the New England Journal of Medicine, suggested that dance can improve brain health. Researchers examined the effect that different 11 types of physical activities on elderly participants. These involved cycling, swimming, tennis and golf. Only dancing lowered the participant's risk of dementia.

Dance is also found to be associated with one's emotions. The facial expressions, body gestures and postures not only help in expressing one's emotions but to be able to generate positive emotions. An individual feels sense of achievement and confidence which further improves the mental health. The dancers become more emotionally intelligent. The present research has also found that dancers are less neurotic than the non-dancers. It means that dancers can better regulate their moods and emotions. Dance also provides an opportunity to ventilate one's feelings in the form of catharsis. It is also said 'letting loose' helps in reducing the level of stress and anxiety also.

Dance can also help in improvement of the interpersonal relationships. As found in the present research also, the people involved in dancing develop more extraversion among them, due to which they interact more with others and are more sociable. The dancers develop betters ways of dealing with others and dealing with their relationships. It improves their social life. When the social aspects are strengthens, it improves the other aspects as well.

Through dance, one can also connect with own body. One can directly express himself through body with the dance being the most fundamental of arts. It can open interesting doorways to our psyche by understanding the relationship with body. Dance includes another important element that is music. The individual listens to the music and to the words/lyrics. All these elements helps in becoming aware of ourselves, our limitations and our movement preferences, our fear of non-verbal expressions degree of confidence in attitude and monotony of moving in conditioned way. All of these factors will impact our relationship with environment and our personality and behavior.

The findings, published in the New England Journal of Medicine suggested that Dancing on a regular basis is associated with a 76 percent reduction in dementia risk. It was said that if an individual does not find exercise to be an enjoyable activity, the person will not get involved in it. Dancing is thus an exercise which involves entertainment, rhythm, music. The enjoyable involvement in dance can trigger the release of feel good hormones like serotonin and endorphins.

Some other research works have supported the findings of the present work. Arpita C. (2013) studied that Dance increases total body movement, which helps to improve circulatory, respiratory, skeletal and muscular systems. It has a positive effect on physical health as well as mental and emotional welling. Mastura J., Mardian S. and Haizan T. (2015) studied the effect of a 12 week low intensity dance exercise intervention in the treatment of hostility subscale, anxiety subscale and depression subscale among overweight women working in Malaysia. The result concluded that the dance intervention had contributed positively to physical health as well as psychological well-being. Kiraly, Urban, Griffiths & Demetrrics studied that dancing is a popular form of physical exercise and studies have shown that dancing can decrease anxiety, increase self-esteem and improve psychological wellbeing.

The dance and therapeutic dance have also been found helpful in controlling various mental ailments be it depression, anxiety, dementia, attention deficit hyperactivity disorder etc.

Sobline, Teresa, Sissy & Roleyn (2014) studied the effect of dance movement therapy on health related psychological problems. Results suggested that dance is effective for increasing quality of life and decreasing clinical symptoms such as depression and anxiety. According to a study published in Frontiers in Human Neuroscience, "dancing may be a better form of exercise than traditional fitness training when it comes to slowing the signs of aging. This is because of the added mental challenges required, which include remembering dance steps. Holding the partner in right way, executing turns, recognizing the beat and synchronizing movement with music, all of these activities are mentioned to as "sensorimotor demands". They relate to bodily activity or movement triggered by sensory as well as motor impulses."

Gronlund, Renck & Weileull (2005) studied a short-term dance movement therapy for two young boys with symptoms related to Attention Deficit Hyperactivity Disorder (ADHD). The DMT has promoted a positive change to a certain extent. DMT provided in paired groups for a minimum of ten weeks will (1) improve the motor function and (2) reduce the behavioural and emotional symptoms of boys with ADHD.

Another study at the University of Illinois at Chicago examined a Latin ballroom dance program for older sedentary adults. The senior dancers disclosed improvements in memory, focus and attention, through the programme. The memory and thinking of participants had improved after the 10-month long dancing session. The same study concluded that "Age related degeneration in brain structure and cognitive impairment may be mitigated with physical activity, especially dance. This is because dance requires more than just motor skills so there is more thinking associated with it."

Conclusion

In the present research, dance has been beneficial for neuroticism factor of personality, physical health, mental health and level of anxiety. The other personality factors such as extraversion, agreeableness, openness to experience and conscientiousness have not been found to be affected by dance movement therapy. The minimum duration dance training was kept three months as the inclusion criteria in the present research. The average dance training duration for the 60 dance trainees in the dance trainee (DT) group was 5 months. One reason for not getting significant result may be the duration of dance training. The dance training might have long term effect on some other variables. The average 5-month training duration might not be sufficient for the dance to show its positive effects on the psychological aspects of an individual. The dance training duration can be increased in further researches to get a better picture of dance training.

The Dance Movement Therapy intervention was also planned for 4 weeks. DMT has also shown positive effect on extraversion also which was not significant with the dance training. It is recommended for further researches to plan dance-movement therapy sessions for longer duration than four-weeks for getting better results.

Dance has been found to be having benefits on the physical and mental health. It also lowers level of neuroticism. It also helps in lowering the level of anxiety. The dance movement therapy can have positive effect on making individual more extraverted, excitement seeking, gregarious, assertive and motives them to involve more with the external world.

CHAPTER-5

IMPLICATIONS, SUGGESTIONS AND LIMITATIONS

The outcomes of a research must be understood and the knowledge obtained through the findings should subsequently be used for the benefit of the society at large. This chapter presents some implications based on the present research findings. Implications refer to how the findings of a particular research can be important for practitioners, policy decision makers, for theory builders of a discipline and for the future researchers. This chapter has also listed certain suggestions for the future researchers which will be useful in framing research objectives, selecting relevant variables and methodology for further researches. No research can be free from any limitations due to constraints of the time, available funds and the manpower. Some limitations of this research are also discussed in this chapter.

The present research has studied the effect of dance training and gender on personality, psychophysical health and anxiety. It has been found that dance affects certain dimensions of personality, anxiety and psychophysical health of an individual. The effect of Dance Movement Therapy as an intervention has also been studied and found to be effective. The use of various arts forms as therapeutic interventions are being used. The use of dance as a form of physical exercise, recreational activity and as a psychotherapeutic alternative is recommended for the treatment of various mental health issues.

5.1 IMPLICATIONS

Certain benefits of dance and dance movement therapy have been discussed along with the implications of this research for the benefit of the society.

- **Promotion of Dance Movement Therapy:** On the basis of the findings of the present research, there is a need to increase the use of Dance Movement Therapy as a part of psychotherapeutic intervention. Looking at the demographic profile at global and national level, it has been found that youth have suffered from the issues of anxiety and other related mental health issues. It is recommended that the psychotherapists, psychologists, mental health practitioners can be trained on the use of Dance Movement Therapy so that skilled dance movement therapist can be available to use dance movement therapy as a therapeutic intervention to control the level of anxiety, stress and depression among the general population.

- **Skilled and Competent DMT Professionals:** Availability of trained professions who can use dance as a form of psychotherapy is also a challenge. More training workshops are needed for preparing a pool of competent and skilled DMT professionals. The training programs need to be supported by allocating funds through various governmental schemes to make these workshops affordable to the aspiring DMT professionals.

- **Inclusion in Personality Development Programmes:** Dance training also helps in improving some personality dimensions such as extraversion and neuroticism among adolescents. Dance Training as a form of physical exercise can be a part of personality development programmes. In this research it is found that dance is helpful in enhancing extrovert behaviour of individual which means the one who practices dance on regular basis makes an individual more expressive, assertive who can communication oneself with others which leads to increase in confidence level in the person.

- **Budget in Health Policy:** There is a need to promote use of various art therapies in clinical settings. Sufficient budget need to be allocated to the institutes and professionals who provide various forms of art therapy including dance training and dance movement therapy. Health policy makers must include dance which is a form of physical exercises which not only affects physical health related parameters but it also helps in improving emotions, moods, personality and also contributes positively at the interpersonal relationship fronts.

- **Mental Health Issues:** It has been established in the present and many other researches that dance helps in reducing anxiety level. Researchers have shown that when we perform dance our body releases endorphins and this hormone reduces depression, anxiety and stress. In day to day life most of the people suffer with anxiety and related symptoms. There are many reasons behind increase in anxiety level such as stress at work, stress from school, financial stress, stress in personal life for example stress in marriage, stress from an emotional trauma like death of loved one, stress from serious medical illness.

Sometimes even it becomes difficult for a doctor to find reason behind increased anxiety. A psychologist and dance movement therapist must work together so that the level of anxiety in an individual can be controlled. It is important to control impulsivity, anger and other emotional imbalance related issues. The use of DMT can be used to control intense negative emotions, impulsivity, mood disorders and other related issues which are a potential cause for substance abuse, suicidal ideation, suicidal attempts and depression. It also hampers one's interpersonal relationships.

- **Obesity and Chronic Illnesses:** Obesity is a major cause for many other chronic illnesses. The present and many other researchers have concluded that dance is very beneficial for our psychophysical health. The use of dance as a form of physical exercise must be a part of various personality development programs. It is considered as a type of exercise. Nowadays, importance of Zumba which is type of dance has been increased for improving physical fitness. Apart from this importance of Aerobics dance form, Bollywood dance in physical fitness has been increased. Dance not only helps in reducing our body weight and physical fitness but it also helps us to be mentally fit. Dance as a form of exercise is useful in controlling obesity and other health and fitness related issues.

- **Physical Health Improvement:** Researches show that along with physical health it is very important to be mentally fit in one's life. It is should always be taken into consideration that how we think? How we feel? How we act in different situation which shows our mental health. With the help of dance, the mental health of peoples of different age groups; children, adults or senior citizens, their health and cognitive abilities can be improved. Dance enhances release of Dopamine and Endorphins in our body and these neurotransmitters are responsible for our pleasure feeling and happiness. Dance is not only beneficial for children and teenagers but is also beneficial for adults and old aged person. A study conducted on persons belonging to age group of 65-91 years in North Dakota reveals that dance improves mood and cognitive health of elderly persons as well. Dance therapy is recommended for the people who are suffering from obesity, depression, stress or anxiety. A dance class or exercise class or even in performing dance is also beneficial for healthy living.

- **Hospitals, Schools and Workplace Settings:** A counsellor in schools should organise dance sessions for the cognitive development, social skills and for overall personality development. Psychologist should organise dance session for the patients in hospitals who are suffering from any disease or illness and admitted in hospitals since a long time so their disease related anxiety can be reduced if it prevails in them. Dance sessions need to be open not only for person having physical illness but also for the healthy people who want to get benefitted by the dance and movement therapy. The companies should also organise dance sessions 1 or 2 times in a month for their employees with the help of psychologist who are trained in dance movement therapy. Also, the dance therapy should be given in old-age home, orphanage, deaf and dumb schools and NGOs etc so there mental and physical health can be improved.

- **Fostering Creativity & Innovation:** Dance is not only like performing high energy movements on high beats but it can also be soft and relaxing. We can say that dance is form of expression. From ancient times people of different communities and tribes expresses their thoughts and sentiments though dance. It is seen that dance enhances our creativity level. Dance and DMT can be used to foster creativity.

- **Fun Learning:** In academic settings also, dance can be incorporated as a fun way of learning. The use of dance along with the academic content can be used in creative way for children and specially-abled children so that their learning experiences can be improved and eased.

5.2 SUGGESTIONS

- The present research has studied the effect of dance on personality, anxiety and health. Some other variables can also be selected as dependent variables such as Creativity, Memory, Emotional Intelligence, Body Image, Interpersonal relationships, level of concentration, attention, cognitive functioning, Well-being etc.

- It is suggested that the future researchers focus on studies the difference in the effect of specific dance forms. Different groups can be provided specific dance forms and the comparison of these dance forms can also be planned.

- The sample consisted of the population in the age group of 18-30 years only. The further research must select sample from the other age groups i.e. children, middle age, elderly people so that the effect of dance on their health and other variables can also be understood.
- The present research has been conducted in the urban settings. Future research can be planned on the rural population also.
- Some specific studies are suggested for the dancers, choreographers who have been involved in dance since more than 5-10 years so that the effect of long term involvement in dance can also be understood. Comparative studies of dancers and non-dancers on various parameters would be more precisely understood when the sample of dancers has undergone long-term training/involvement in dance.
- There is a need to conduct researches which compare Indian and Western dance forms and its effect on the physical health, mental health, personality and other psychological variables. The research studying the effect of Kathak, Bharatnatyam, Kuchipudi and other classical dance forms on the various psychological parameters such as moods, emotional regulation, communication, level of confidence, self esteem, cognitive functioning etc can also be conducted.
- The Intervention Model used in this research has been implemented for four weeks. It is recommended that the future researchers could increase the duration of dance movement therapy intervention to gain a better output after the intervention.
- Some other population groups can also be provided dance movement therapy. The future researchers can conduct studies on the children, elderly population, juvenile delinquents, individuals/children who have suicidal ideations/attempts history and the patients of some specific diseases. The use of dance and other art forms as a way of obtaining deeper information need to be studied.

5.3 LIMITATIONS

- The present research has certain limitations related to the sample selected. The sample consisted of 120 adolescents only. The increase in the sample size would help in getting more generalized findings.
- There were some geographical constraints in the sample which is taken only from Udaipur while the sample from outside Udaipur can also be taken. For a more generalized findings, a research on the wider geographical area could be conducted.
- The sample taken was of the persons of the age group between 18-30 groups while the people from the others age group below or above this age group can also be studies to the effect of dance and dance movement therapy on various psychological variables. The findings of this research are applicable on the adolescents only.
- The intervention of dance movement therapy was also conducted on 20 adolescents; with 10 adolescents in each group i.e. control group and experimental group.

CHAPTER-6

SUMMARY

The title of the present research is 'Personality & Psychophysical Health in relation to Dance Training: A Therapeutic Intervention of Dance Movement Therapy' On the basis of the review of literature, some major **research gaps** were identified. There are fewer researches comparing the psychological profiles of dancers and non-dancers. The researches focusing the effect of Dance and Movement Therapy in Indian contests are available but are limited in number to develop a comprehensive picture.

The following research objectives and hypotheses were framed:

6.1 OBJECTIVES

1. To study the effect of Dance Training on personality (Openness, Conscientiousness, Extraversion, Agreeableness and Neuroticism), level of anxiety & psychophysical health
2. To study the effect of gender on an individual's personality, level of anxiety & psychophysical health
3. To study the interaction effect of gender (male & female) and dance training (dance trainee & non dance trainee) on personality, level of anxiety & psychophysical health
4. To prepare an intervention model based on Dance Movement Therapy
5. Therapeutic intervention of Dance Movement Therapy to study its effect on personality, level of anxiety & psychophysical health

6.2 HYPOTHESES

1. There is no difference between the personality of Dance Trainee and Non-Dance Trainee.
2. There is no difference between the psychophysical health of Dance Trainee and Non-Dance Trainee.
3. There is no difference between the level of anxiety of Dance Trainee and Non-Dance Trainee.

4. There is no difference between the personality of Males and Females.

5. There is no difference between the psychophysical health of Males and Females.

6. There is no difference between the level of anxiety of Males and Females.

7. There is no effect of therapeutic use of dance movement therapy on personality, psychophysical health and anxiety.

6.3 VARIABLES

Dance Training and Gender have been selected as the independent variables for the present research. Dance Training has two categories Dance Trainee and Non-Dance Trainee. Gender also has two categories Male and Female.

The following three variables were selected as dependents variables for the present research.

a. Personality – Big five traits

(Openness, Conscientiousness, Extraversion, Agreeableness and Neuroticism)

b. Psychophysical Health (Mental and Physical health)

c. Anxiety

6.4 RESEARCH DESIGN

The present research was conducted in two phases. In the first phase, the researcher collected data from the sample of 120 adolescents selected as per the factorial design shown below. In the second phase, the researcher conducted dance-movement therapy on 20 adolescents divided in two groups; one control and one experimental group.

Phase I

A total sample of 120 adolescents was selected as per the 2x2 factorial design.

Table 6.1 : 2x2 factorial design (Phase-I)

	Dance Trainee (B_1)	**Non-Dance Trainee (B_2)**	**Total**
Male (A_1)	A_1B_1 (N=30)	A_1B_2 (N=30)	60
Female (A_2)	A_2B_1 (N=30)	A_2B_2 (N=30)	60
Total	60	60	120

Phase II

An intervention model based on the dance-movement therapy principles and techniques was prepared by the researcher. This intervention model was used by the researcher to provide dance-movement therapy to selected adolescents in Phase-II of the research. A sample of 20 adolescents was selected randomly from 60 adolescents from Phase-I. A Before-After Two group Control-Experimental Design was used for the Phase-II therapeutic sessions.

Table 6.2: Before-After Two Groups Design (Phase II)

Group	Pre-test	Intervention	Post-test
Control Group (N=10)	• Personality • Psychophysical health • Anxiety	No Intervention	• Personality • Psychophysical health • Anxiety
Experimental Group (N=10)	• Anxiety Personality • Psychophysical health • Anxiety	Intervention (Dance Movement Therapy)	• Personality • Psychophysical health • Anxiety

The locale of the present study was confined to Udaipur district of Rajasthan. The sample was selected from the different Dance Institutes of Udaipur. The sample of non-dancers is also taken from Udaipur district.

Table 6.3 : Psychological tests/tools used for Data Collection

VARIABLE	NAME OF THE TEST/SCALE	AUTHOR
Personality	Big Five personality test	Costa & McCrae, 1992
Anxiety	Sinha Anxiety Scale	D. N. Sinha, 1976
Psychophysical health	P.G.I. Health Questionnaire	S K Verma, 1971

Mean, S.D. and ANOVA were used for analyzing the data obtained in Phase-I and paired sample t-test was used to compare the control and experimental group in Phase-II.

6.5 FINDINGS

The summary of main findings of the present research has been given below.

- 72.5% of the respondents are falling in either very high or high category on the level of neuroticism whereas only 26.6% respondents are falling in the normal category on Neuroticism. 77% have very high to high to normal levels of extraversion. 65% of the respondents have scored either very low or low on the Openness to Experience dimension of Big-five personality traits. 67.49% of respondents are low on Agreeableness. On the level of Conscientiousness, 65% of the respondents have scored very low to low.

- Male respondents are more neurotic than female respondents. There is no significantly effect of Dance Training on Neuroticism. The interaction effect of gender and dance training on the level of neuroticism has been found significant at .01 levels.

- Among the four groups, the male dancers group has shown higher level of extraversion whereas the male non-dancers group has shown lowest level of extraversion. The dance trainees exhibited more Extraversion than the non-dance trainees. The main effect of gender on Extraversion was not found significant. The interaction effect of Gender and Dance Training on Extraversion was found significant at 0.05 levels.

- There is no effect of Dance Training on Agreeableness, Openness and Conscientiousness. There is no effect of Gender on Agreeableness, Openness and Conscientiousness. There is no interaction effect of Dance Training and Gender on Agreeableness, Openness and Conscientiousness.

- The Anxiety score of Dance Trainee group is less than the Non-Dance Trainee group. The female respondents have more Anxiety than male respondents, however, this difference is not found to be statistically significant. The interaction effect of gender and dance training on Anxiety was also not found to be significant.

- The Dance Trainee respondents have better physical health and mental health than the Non-Dance Trainee respondents. The female respondents have better Physical and mental health than the male respondents. The interaction effect of Gender and Dance Training on both Physical and mental health was also found significant at 0.01 levels.

- The dance movement therapy intervention has been beneficial for neuroticism and extraversion factors of personality, physical health, mental health and level of anxiety. The other personality factors such as agreeableness, openness to experience and conscientiousness have not been found to be affected by dance movement therapy.

There is a need to increase the use of Dance Movement Therapy as a part of psychotherapeutic intervention. Availability of trained professions who can use dance as a form of psychotherapy is also a challenge. More training workshops are needed for preparing a pool of competent and skilled DMT professionals. Dance training is recommended to included in Personality Development Programmes, more funds need to be allocated for organizing workshops for various art therapies. The use of art therapy is recommended to treat both mental Health Issues. DMT can also be used for physical health Improvement. It is suggested that the future researchers should select the dancers who have been trained in dance for longer duration, at least one-year dance training.

REFERENCES

A Specialized Dance/Movement Therapy Assessment and Proposed Plan for Addressing the Physical and Emotional Well-being of Line Workers. (2020). Retrieved March 3, 2021, from https://digitalcommons.lesley.edu/cgi/viewcontent.cgi?article=1354&context=expressive_theses

Akandere, M., & Demir, B. (2011). The effect of dance over depression. Coll. Antropol., 35 (3), 651-656.

Annesi, H., Merali, Z., Poulter, M.O., & Hayley, S. (2005). Changes in depressed mood associated with 10 weeks of moderate cardiovascular exercise in formerly sedentary adults. Psychological Reports, 96, 855 — 862.

Australian Psychological Society (2010). Evidence-based psychological interventions in the treatment of mental disorders: A literature review (3rded.). The Australian Psychological Society Ltd.

Aweto H. A., Owoeye O. B., Akinbo S. R., Onabajo A. A. (2012). Effects of dance movement therapy on selected cardiovascular parameters and estimated maximum oxygen consumption in hypertensive patients. Nig. Q. J. Hosp. Med. 22, 125–129.

Barton, E. J. (2011). Movement and mindfulness: a formative evaluation of dance/ movement and yoga therapy program with participants experiencing severe mental illness. American Journal of Dance Therapy, Vol 33, Issue 2, Page No. 157-181

Barton, E. J. (2011). Movement and mindfulness: a formative evaluation of dance/ movement and yoga therapy program with participants experiencing severe mental illness. American Journal of Dance Therapy, Vol 33, Issue 2, Page No. 157-181

Behrends, A. and Muller, S. and Dziobek, I. (2012). Moving in and out of synchrony : A concept for a new intervention fostering empathy through interactional movement and dance. Vol 39, Issue 2, Page No. 107-116. Retrieved from http://scholar.cnki.net/ detail/sjestemp_U/SJ

Behrends, A. and Muller, S. and Dziobek, I. (2012). Moving in and out of synchrony: A concept for a new intervention fostering empathy through interactional movement and dance. Vol 39, Issue 2, Page No. 107-116. Retrieved from http://scholar.cnki.net/ detail/sjestemp_U/SJ

Bentzen, M. (2015). Dances of connection: Neuroaffective development in clinical work with attachment. Body, Movement and Dance in Psychotherapy, 10, 211–226.

Bohlmeijer E., Prenger R., Taal E., Cuijpers P. (2010). The effects of mindfulness-based stress reduction therapy on mental health of adults with a chronic medical disease: a meta-analysis. J. Psychosom. Res. 68, 539–544.

Bojner-Horwitz, E. (2004). 243-Dance/Movement Therapy And Changes In Stress-Related Hormones: A Study Of Fibromyalgia Patients. In , & , *Journal of Psychosomatic Research* (Vols. 56, Issues 6, p. 633). https://doi.org/10.1016/j.jpsychores.2004.04.232

Bräuninger I. (2012a). The efficacy of dance movement therapy group on improvement of quality of life: a randomized controlled trial. Arts Psychother. 39, 296–303. 10.1016/j.aip.2012.03.008

Brauninger, I. (2012). The efficiency of dance movement therapy group on improvement of quality of life : A randomized control trial. Vol 39, Issue 4, Page No. 293-303. Retrieved from www.journals.elsevier.com

Brauninger, I. (2012). The efficiency of dance movement therapy group on improvement of quality of life: A randomized control trial. Vol 39, Issue 4, Page No. 293-303. Retrieved from www.journals.elsevier.com

Brauninger, I. (2014, May). *Dance movement therapy with the elderly: An international Internet* .. researchgate.Net. Retrieved March 3, 2021, from https://www.tandfonline.com/doi/abs/10.1080/17432979.2014.914977

Brooklyn, L. Exploring dance/movement therapy to treat women with posttraumatic stress disorder. Retrieved from http://www1.uwindsor.ca/criticalsocialwork/ dancemovement therapy

Brooklyn, L. Exploring dance/movement therapy to treat women with posttraumatic stress disorder. Retrieved from http://www1.uwindsor.ca/ criticalsocialwork/dancemovement therapy

Burgess G., Grogan S., Burwitz L. (2006). Effects of a 6-week aerobic dance intervention on body image and physical self-perceptions in adolescent girls. Body Image 3, 57–66. 10.1016/j.bodyim.2005.10.005

Campbell-Sills, L., Barlow, D. H., Brown, T. A., & Hofmann, S. G. (2006). Effects of suppression and acceptance on emotional responses of individuals with anxiety and mood disorders. Behaviour Research and Therapy 44, 1251–1263.

Carlson E. Burger B. and Touranen P. (2018). Dance like someone is watching: A social Realtions Model study of Music-Induced Movement. Retrieved from https://journals.sagepub.com/doi/10.1177/2059204318807846

Chatterjee, A. (2013). The Therapeutic Value of Indian Classical, Folk and Innovative Dance Forms. Rupkatha Journal on Interdisciplinary Studies in Humanities Vol. V, No. 1, 2013. Retrieved from http://rupkatha.com/the-therapeutic-value-of-indian-classical-folk-and-innovative-dance-forms/

Chatterjee, A. (2013). The Therapeutic Value of Indian Classical, Folk and Innovative Dance Forms. Rupkatha Journal on Interdisciplinary Studies in Humanities Vol. V, No. 1, 2013. Retrieved from http://rupkatha.com/the-therapeutic-value-of-indian-classical-folk-and-innovative-dance-forms/

Colucci, J. Dance Therapy and Relaxation Therapy: Effects on Anxiety. Saint Anselm College, Dept. of Psychology. Retrieved from http://www.anselm.edu/internet/ psych/ theses/seniors2002/colucci/#abstract

Colucci, J. Dance Therapy and Relaxation Therapy: Effects on Anxiety. Saint Anselm College, Dept. of Psychology. Retrieved from http://www.anselm.edu/internet/ psych/ theses/seniors2002/colucci/# abstract

Corteville, M. K. (2009). Dance Your Way to Communication: Dance Movement Therapy to Increase Self-Esteem, Poor Body Image, and Communication Skills in High School Females. Student Counselling & Personal Services Commons. Retrieved from http://digitalcommons.brockport.edu/edc_theses/21/

Corteville, M. K. (2009). Dance Your Way to Communication: Dance Movement Therapy to Increase Self-Esteem, Poor Body Image, and Communication Skills in High School Females. Student Counselling & Personal Services Commons. Retrieved from http://digitalcommons.brockport.edu/ edc_theses/21/

Crain, C. & McLoughlin, J. & Eisenhart, M. (1983). The Social and Physical Effects of a 10-Week Dance Program on Educable Mentally Retarded Adolescents. Education and Training of the Mentally Retarded. Retrieved from http://www.jstor.org/stable/ 23877241?seq=1#page_scan_tab_contents

Crain, C. & McLoughlin, J. & Eisenhart, M. (1983). The Social and Physical Effects of a 10-Week Dance Program on Educable Mentally Retarded Adolescents. Education and Training of the Mentally Retarded. Retrieved from http://www.jstor.org/stable/23877241?seq=1#page_scan_tab_ contents

Cross K., Flores R., Butterfield J., Blackman M., Lee S. (2012). The effect of passive listening versus active observation of music and dance performances on memory recognition and mild to moderate depression in cognitively impaired older adults. Psychol. Rep. 111, 413–423. 10.2466/10.02.13.PR0.111.5.413-423

Dance Movement Therapy | Therapy Types | Zencare. 2021. *Dance Movement Therapy | Therapy Types | Zencare*. [online] Available at: <https://zencare.co/therapy-type/dance-movement-therapy> [Accessed 2 March 2021].

DANCE MOVEMENT THERAPY AS REHABILITATION PROCESS FOR WOMEN WITH FALLS HISTORY. (2015). In, & , *The Gerontologist* (Vols. 55, Issue _2, p. 719). https://doi.org///doi.org/10.1093/geront/gnv358.03

Dance Therapy and Relaxation Therapy: Effects on Anxiety. Saint Anselm College, Department of Psychology

Daytom, E. F. (2010). The Creative Use of Dance/Movement Therapy Processes to Transform Intrapersonal Conflicts Associated with Sexual Trauma in Women. Portland State University. Retrieved from http://pdxscholar.library.pdx.edu/ cgi/viewcontent.cgi? article=1385&context=open_access_etds

Daytom, E. F. (2010). The Creative Use of Dance/Movement Therapy Processes to Transform Intrapersonal Conflicts Associated with Sexual Trauma in Women. Portland State University. Retrieved from http:// pdxscholar.library.pdx.edu/cgi/viewcontent.cgi? article=1385&context=open_access_etds

Dempsey, M. (2009). Dance/movement therapy as an effective clinical intervention to decreases anxiety and support the recover process. In S. Brooke (Ed.). The use of creative therapies with chemical dependency issues (pp. 162-173). Springfield, IL. Charles C. Thomas Publisher Ltd.

Dr. Rainbow, H.T. H. (2014). Effects of dance/movement therapy on the disease symptoms in breast cancer patients undergoing radiotherapy. The HKU Scholars Hub. Retrieved from http://hub.hku.hk/handle/10722/197779

Dr. Rainbow, H.T. H. (2014). Effects of dance/movement therapy on the disease symptoms in breast cancer patients undergoing radiotherapy. The HKU Scholars Hub. Retrieved from http://hub.hku.hk/handle/10722/197779

Dulicai, D. & Hill, E.S. (2007). Expressive movement. In Low-cost approaches to promote physical and mental health (Part 3). 177 — 200. DOI: 10.1007/0-387-36899-x9

Effects of dance on anxiety (1990). American Journal of Dance Therapy, Volume 12, Issue 1, Pages 19-25

Elizabeth, A. and Gray, L. (2011). The Body Remembers: Dance/Movement Therapy with an Adult Survivor of Torture. American Journal of Dance Therapy, Vol 23, Issue 1, Page No. 29-43. Retrieved from http://link.springer.com/article/10.1023/A% 3A1010780306585#page-1

Elizabeth, A. and Gray, L. (2011). The Body Remembers: Dance/Movement Therapy with an Adult Survivor of Torture. American Journal of Dance Therapy, Vol 23, Issue 1, Page No. 29-43. Retrieved from http://link.springer.com/article/10.1023/A% 3A1010780306585#page-1

Ferreri L., Bigand E. and Bugaiska A (2015). The positive effect of music on source memory. Retrieved from http://journals.sagepub.com/doi/abs/ 10.1177/1029864915604684

Five-factor model of personality and job satisfaction: A meta-analysis (2002). Journal of Applied Psychology, Vol 87(3), Pages 530-541. Retrieved from http://dx.doi.org/10.1037/0021-9010.87.3.530

Gallagher, S. (2005). How the body shapes the mind. New York: Oxford University Press.

Gammo M. E. (2009). Dance as Therapy for Individuals with Parkinson Disease. Retrieved from www.ncbi.nlm.nih.gov/pmc/articles/pmc2780534

Gammo M. E. (2009). Dance as Therapy for Individuals with Parkinson Disease. Retrieved from www.ncbi.nlm.nih.gov/pmc/articles/pmc2780534

Gronlund, E. and Renck, B. and Weibull, J. (2005). Dance/Movement Therapy as an Alternative Treatment for Young Boys Diagnosed as ADHD: A Pilot Study, American Journal of Dance therapy, Vol 27, Issue 2, Page No. 63-85. Retrieved from http://www.researchgate.net/publication/227238006_DanceMovement_Therapy_as_an_Alternative_Treatment_for_Young_Boys_Diagnosed_as_ADHD_A_Pilot_Study

Gronlund, E. and Renck, B. and Weibull, J. (2005). Dance/Movement Therapy as an Alternative Treatment for Young Boys Diagnosed as ADHD: A Pilot Study, American Journal of Dance Therapy, Vol 27, Issue 2, Page No. 63-85. Retrieved from http://www.researchgate.net/publication/ 227238006_DanceMovement_Therapy_as_an_Alternative_Treatment_for_Young_Boys_Diagnosed_as_ADHD_A_Pilot_Study

Hanna, J. L. (2011). Dancing for health. Body Movement and Dance in Psychotherapy: An International Journal for Theory, Research and Practice, 6 (1), 77-80

http://www.cheshireeast.gov.uk/social_care_and_health/health_advice/physical_health.aspx

Jeong, Y. J.A. and Hong, S. C. and Lee, M. S. & Park, M. and Kim, Y. K. & Suh, C. M. (2005). Dance Movement Therapy improves emotional responses and modulates neurohormones in adolescents with mild depression, International Journal of Neuroscience, Vol 115, Issue 12. Retrieved from http://www.tandfonline.com/doi/abs/10.1080/00207450590958574 #.Vfv0jNKqqko

Jeong, Y. J.A. and Hong, S. C. and Lee, M. S. & Park, M. and Kim, Y. K. & Suh, C. M. (2005). Dance Movement Therapy improves emotional responses and modulates neurohormones in adolescents with mild depression, International Journal of Neuroscience, Vol 115, Issue 12. Retrieved from http://www.tandfonline.com/doi/abs/10.1080/00207450590958574

Jojhar, M. & Shah M. & Taha (2015). Effect of Low Intensity Dance Exercise: Hostility, Anxiety and Depression among Sedentary Overweight Women in Malaysia, Universal Journal of Psychology Vol. 3(3), Dept. of Social Science, University of Tenaga National, Malaysia. Retrieved from http://www.hrpub. org/journals/article_info.php ?aid=2512

Jojhar, M. & Shah M. & Taha (2015). Effect of Low Intensity Dance Exercise: Hostility, Anxiety and Depression among Sedentary Overweight Women in Malaysia, Universal Journal of Psychology Vol. 3(3), Dept. of Social Science, University of Tenaga National, Malaysia. Retrieved from http://www.hrpub.org/journals/article_info.php?aid=2512

Karpati, F. J. & Giacosa, C. & Foster, N. E.V. & Virginia B & Penhune & Hyde, Krista L. Annals of the New York Academy of Sciences Volume 1337 Dance and the brain: a review (2015). Retrieved from http://onlinelibrary.wiley.com/doi/ 101111/nyas. 12632/abstract

Karpati, F. J. & Giacosa, C. & Foster, N. E.V. & Virginia B & Penhune & Hyde, Krista L. Annals of the New York Academy of Sciences Volume 1337 Dance and the brain: a review (2015). Retrieved from http://onlinelibrary.wiley.com/ doi/101111/nyas. 12632/abstract

Kaufman, Gabrielle. Dance Movement Therapy. Retrieved from http://www.gabrielle kaufman.com/Gabrielle_Kaufman/Dance_Movement_Therapy

Kaufman, Gabrielle. Dance Movement Therapy. Retrieved from http://www.gabriellekaufman.com/Gabrielle_Kaufman/Dance_Movement _Therapy

Kendra C., What Is Positive Thinking? Retrieved from http://psychology.about. com/od/PositivePsychology/f/positive-thinking.htm

Kendra C., What Is Positive Thinking? Retrieved from http://psychology.about. com/od/PositivePsychology/f/positive-thinking.htm

Kiepe, Sophie M. & Stockigt & Keil, T. (2012). Effects of dance therapy and ballroom dances on physical and mental illnesses: A systematic review, Vol 39, Issue 5, Page No. 404- 411. Retrieved from http://www.sciencedirect.com/science/ article/pii/S0197455612000998

Kiepe, Sophie M. & Stockigt & Keil, T. (2012). Effects of dance therapy and ballroom dances on physical and mental illnesses: A systematic review, Vol 39, Issue 5, Page No. 404- 411. Retrieved from http://www.sciencedirect.com/science/article/pii/S0197455612000 998

Koch S. C. (2007). The Arts in Psychotherapy, Vol 36, Issue 4, Page No. 340-349. Retrieved from www.sciencedirect.com

Koch S. C. (2007). The Arts in Psychotherapy, Vol 36, Issue 4, Page No. 340-349. Retrieved from www.sciencedirect.com

Koch, S. & Kunj, T. & Lykou, S. & Cruz, R. (2014). The joy dance Specific effects of a single dance intervention on psychiatric patients with depression, Vol. 41 Issue 1. Retrieved from http://www.adta.org/Resources/Documents/Koch%20-%20The %20joy%20dance%20study.pdf

Koch, S. & Kunj, T. & Lykou, S. & Cruz, R. (2014). The joy dance Specific effects of a single dance intervention on psychiatric patients with depression, Vol. 41 Issue 1. Retrieved from http://www.adta.org/Resources/Documents/Koch%20-%20The %20joy%20dance%20study.pdf

Koshlan, L. & Wilson, J. & Wittakar B. (2004). PEACE Through Dance/Movement: Evaluating a Violence Prevention Program, American Journal of Dance Therapy, Vol 26, Issue 2, Page No. 69-90. Retrieved from http://adta.org/Resources/Documents/ Koshland%20Wittaker%202004.pdf

Koshlan, L. & Wilson, J. & Wittakar B. (2004). PEACE Through Dance/Movement: Evaluating a Violence Prevention Program, American Journal of Dance Therapy, Vol 26, Issue 2, Page No. 69-90. Retrieved from http://adta.org/Resources/Documents/ Koshland%20Wittaker%202004.pdf

Leventhan, Fern and Chang, Meg (1991). Dance Movement Therapy with battered women : A Paradigm of Action, American Journal of Dance Therapy, Vol 13, Issue 2, Page No. 131-145. Retrieved from http://link.springer.com/article/10.1007/BF00844142#page-1

Leventhan, Fern and Chang, Meg (1991). Dance Movement Therapy with battered women : A Paradigm of Action, American Journal of Dance Therapy, Vol 13, Issue 2, Page No. 131-145. Retrieved from http://link.springer.com/article/10.1007/BF00844142#page-1

Maraz A, Király O, Urbán R, Griffiths MD, Demetrovics Z (2015). Why Do You Dance? Development of the Dance Motivation Inventory (DMI)

Marjolein D. van der Zwaag (2011). The influence of music on mood and performance while driving, Page No. 12-22. Retrieved from http://www.tandfonline.com/doi/full/10.1080/00140139.2011.638403

McGarry, L. M. and Russo, F. A. (2011). Mirroring in Dance/Movement Therapy: Potential mechanisms behind empathy enhancement, Vol 58, Issue 3, Page No. 178-184. Retrieved from http://www.journals.elsevier.com

McGarry, L. M. and Russo, F. A. (2011). Mirroring in Dance/Movement Therapy: Potential mechanisms behind empathy enhancement, Vol 58, Issue 3, Page No. 178-184. Retrieved from http:// www.journals.elsevier.com

Michelle, J. W. (2010). *Challenges faced by movement therapist in terms of recognition of their profession: a project based upon an independent investigation.* Retrieved March 3, 2021, from https://scholarworks.smith.edu/theses/515/

Music Therapy to Reduce Pain and Anxiety in Children with Cancer Undergoing Lumbar Puncture: A Randomized Clinical Trial (2015). Journal of Paediatric Oncology Nursing

Pablo A. Domene, Hannah J. Moir, Elizabeth Pummell, Chris Easton (2015) Salsa dance and Zumba fitness: Acute responses during community-based classes, Retrieved from http://dx.doi.org/10.1016/j.jshs.2015.04.004

Physical Health. Cheshire East council. Retrieved from

Physical Health. Cheshire East council. Retrieved from http://www.cheshireeast.gov.uk/ social_care_and_health/health_advice/physical_health.aspx

Pinniger, R., Thorsteinson, E. B. and Brown, R. F (2013). Tango Dance can reduce distress and insomnia in pupil with Self-Referred Affective symptoms, American Journal of Dance Therapy, Vol 35, Issue 1, Page No. 60-77. Retrieved from http://link.springer.com/article/10.1007/s10465-012-9141-y

Pinniger, R., Thorsteinson, E. B. and Brown, R. F (2013). Tango Dance can reduce distress and insomnia in pupil with Self-Referred Affective symptoms, American Journal of Dance Therapy, Vol 35, Issue 1, Page No. 60-77. Retrieved from http://link.springer.com/article/10.1007/s10465-012-9141-y

Rosenthal, M. (2013). Benefits of Dance Movement Therapy for treating PTSD. Retrieved from http://healmyptsd.com/2013/08/benefits-of-dance-movement-therapy-for-treating-ptsd.html

Rosenthal, M. (2013). Benefits of Dance Movement Therapy for treating PTSD. Retrieved from http://healmyptsd.com/2013/08/benefits-of-dance-movement-therapy-for-treating-ptsd.html

Salgado, R. and Vasconcilos, L.A. (2010). The use of dance in the rehabilitation of a patient with Multiple Sclerosis, American Journal of Dance Therapy, Vol 32, Issue 01, Page No. 53-63. Retrieved from http://link.springer.com/article/10.1007/s10465-010-9087-x

Salgado, R. and Vasconcilos, L.A. (2010). The use of dance in the rehabilitation of a patient with Multiple Sclerosis, American Journal of Dance Therapy, Vol 32, Issue 01, Page No. 53-63. Retrieved from http://link.springer.com/article/10.1007/s10465-010-9087-x

Sandel SL. Integrating dance therapy into treatment. Psychiatric Services. 1975; 26(7):439–41. https://doi.org/10.1176/ps.26.7.439.

Sanderson, P. (2008). The arts, social inclusion and social class: The case of dance, British Educational Research Journal, Vol 34, No. 4. Retrieved from http://onlinelibrary.wiley.com/doi/10.1080/01411920701609349/abstract

Sanderson, P. (2008). The arts, social inclusion and social class: The case of dance, British Educational Research Journal, Vol 34, No. 4. Retrieved from http://onlinelibrary.wiley.com/doi/10.1080/01411920701609349/abstract

Shaw D. Benzio K. (2019). What are some Dance Movement Therapy Techniques Retrieved from https://www.honeylake.clinic/what-are-some-dance-movement-therapy-techniques/

Silberg, D. N. (2012). The Utilization of Movement and Dance to Support Children in the Aftermath of Community Disaster. Retrieved from https://idea.library.drexel.edu/islandora/object/idea%3A3758/datastream/OBJ/download/The_Utilization_of_Movement_and_Dance_to_Support_Children_in_the_Aftermath_of_Community_Disaster.pdf

Silberg, D. N. (2012). The Utilization of Movement and Dance to Support Children in the Aftermath of Community Disaster. Retrieved from https://idea.library.drexel.edu/islandora/object/idea%3A3758/datastream/OBJ/download/The_Utilization_of_Movement_and_Dance_to_Support_Children_in_the_Aftermath_of_Community_Disaster.pdf

Solsvig Shawna L. (2010). Dance/movement therapy and responsive classroom: a theoretical synthesis. Retrieved from http://digitalcommons.colum.edu/cgi/viewcontent.cgi?article=1012&context=theses_dmt

Sport Science Review (2012), Department of Physical Education and Sport Sciences, Aristotle University of Thessaloniki, Greece. Vol 20, Issue 5-6, Pages 105–126

Thachil, A.F. , Mohan, R., & Bhugra, D. (2007). The evidence base of complementary and alternative therapies in depression. Journal of Affective Disorders, 97 (1-3), 23 — 35.

The Effect of Exercise on Body Satisfaction and Self-Esteem as a Function of Gender and Age DOI: 10.1023/A:1007095830095

The effect of low impact dance training on aerobic capacity, submaximal heart rates and body composition of college-aged females (1989). J Sports Med Phys Fitness, Pages 184- 188.

The effects of sport dance on brain connectivity and body intelligence, Journal of Cognitive Psychology DOI: 10.1080/20445911.2016.1177059

The Healing Power of Dance. (2003). Retrieved from http://www.reintegration.com/health/

The joy dance: Specific effects of a single dance intervention on psychiatric patients with depression (2007). The Arts in Psychotherapy, Volume 34, Issue 4, Pages 340–349

The Social and Physical Effects of a 10-Week Dance Program on Educable Mentally Retarded Adolescents. Vol 18, No. 4. Retrieved from http://www.jstor.org/stable/23877241?seq=1#page_scan_tab_contents

The Social and Physical Effects of a 10-Week Dance Program on Educable Mentally Retarded Adolescents. Vol 18, No. 4. Retrieved from http://www.jstor.org/stable/23877241?seq=1#page_scan_tab_contents

Tomas Chamorro-Premuzic, Adrian FTomas, Chamorro, Premuzic, Adrian Furnham (2007). Personality and music: Can traits explain how people use music in everyday life? DOI: 10.1348/000712606X111177

West, M. (2015). Dance your way to better physical and mental health. Retrieved from http://www.naturalnews.com/036481_dancing_physical_health.html

West, M. (2015). Dance your way to better physical and mental health. Retrieved from http://www.naturalnews.com/036481_dancing_physical_health.html

What is Mental Health. Retrieved from http://www.mentalhealth.gov

What is Mental Health. Retrieved from http://www.mentalhealth.gov

What is Positive Thinking? Retrieved from https://leadingpersonality.wordpress.com/2013/ 03/15/what-is-positive-thinking/

What is Positive Thinking? Retrieved from https://leadingpersonality.wordpress.com/2013/ 03/15/what-is-positive-thinking/

Why Do You Dance? Development of the Dance Motivation Inventory (2015). Retrieved from http://dx.doi.org/10.1371/journal.pone.0122866

PERSONAL DATA SHEET

Name : ______________________________

Age : ______________ **Contact No. :** ______________

Gender : ______________________________

Education : ______________________________

Education : ______________________________

School/College : ______________________________

Hobby : ______________________________

Occupation : ______________________________

Dance Trainee [ ] **Non Dance Trainee [ ]** **(Please Tick Appropriate)**

Name of Dance Training Institute : ______________________________

From how long you are taking Dance Training : ______________________________

Aim : ______________________________

NEO™-FFI-3

Item Booklet | Form S–Adult

SELF-REPORT

NEO Five-Factor Inventory-3

Paul T. Costa, Jr., PhD and Robert R. McCrae, PhD

Instructions

Write only where indicated in this Item Booklet. Carefully read all of the instructions before beginning. This questionnaire contains 60 statements. Read each statement carefully. For each statement, fill in the circle with the response that best represents your opinion. Make sure that your answer is in the correct box.

Fill in (SD) if you *strongly disagree* or the statement is definitely false.

Fill in (D) if you *disagree* or the statement is mostly false.

Fill in (N) if you are *neutral* on the statement, if you cannot decide, or if the statement is about equally true and false.

Fill in (A) if you *agree* or the statement is mostly true.

Fill in (SA) if you *strongly agree* or the statement is definitely true.

Note that the responses are numbered in ***rows***.

Example

First five responses from an individual who strongly disagrees with items 1, 2, and 3, and agrees with items 4 and 5.

ENTER ACROSS

1 ● (D) (N) (A) (SA)	2 ● (D) (N) (A) (SA)	3 ● (D) (N) (A) (SA)	4 (SD) (D) (N) ● (SA)	5 (SD) (D) (N) ● (SA)

Fill in only one response for each statement. Respond to all of the statements, making sure that you fill in the correct response. **DO NOT ERASE!** If you need to change an answer, make an "X" through the incorrect response and then fill in the correct response.

Before responding to the statements, turn to the inside of this Item Booklet and enter your name, age, sex, ID number (if any), and today's date.

PAR • 16204 N. Florida Ave. • Lutz, FL 33549 • 1.800.331.8378 • www.parinc.com

9 8 7 6 5 Reorder #RO-6806 Printed in the U.S.A.

ID# ____________

Name ______________________ Age ______ Sex ________ Today's date ____________

1. I am not a worrier.
2. I like to have a lot of people around me.
3. I enjoy concentrating on a fantasy or daydream and exploring all its possibilities, letting it grow and develop.
4. I try to be courteous to everyone I meet.
5. I keep my belongings neat and clean.

6. At times I have felt bitter and resentful.
7. I laugh easily.
8. I think it's interesting to learn and develop new hobbies.
9. At times I bully or flatter people into doing what I want them to.
10. I'm pretty good about pacing myself so as to get things done on time.

11. When I'm under a great deal of stress, sometimes I feel like I'm going to pieces.
12. I prefer jobs that let me work alone without being bothered by other people.
13. I am intrigued by the patterns I find in art and nature.
14. Some people think I'm selfish and egotistical.
15. I often come into situations without being fully prepared.

16. I rarely feel lonely or blue.
17. I really enjoy talking to people.
18. I believe letting students hear controversial speakers can only confuse and mislead them.
19. If someone starts a fight, I'm ready to fight back.
20. I try to perform all the tasks assigned to me conscientiously.

21. I often feel tense and jittery.
22. I like to be where the action is.
23. Poetry has little or no effect on me.
24. I'm better than most people, and I know it.
25. I have a clear set of goals and work toward them in an orderly fashion.

26. Sometimes I feel completely worthless.
27. I shy away from crowds of people.
28. I would have difficulty just letting my mind wander without control or guidance.
29. When I've been insulted, I just try to forgive and forget.
30. I waste a lot of time before settling down to work.

31. I rarely feel fearful or anxious.
32. I often feel as if I'm bursting with energy.
33. I seldom notice the moods or feelings that different environments produce.
34. I tend to assume the best about people.
35. I work hard to accomplish my goals.

36. I often get angry at the way people treat me.
37. I am a cheerful, high-spirited person.
38. I experience a wide range of emotions or feelings.
39. Some people think of me as cold and calculating.
40. When I make a commitment, I can always be counted on to follow through.

41. Too often, when things go wrong, I get discouraged and feel like giving up.
42. I don't get much pleasure from chatting with people.
43. Sometimes when I am reading poetry or looking at a work of art, I feel a chill or wave of excitement.
44. I have no sympathy for beggars.
45. Sometimes I'm not as dependable or reliable as I should be.

46. I am seldom sad or depressed.
47. My life is fast-paced.
48. I have little interest in speculating on the nature of the universe or the human condition.
49. I generally try to be thoughtful and considerate.
50. I am a productive person who always gets the job done.

51. I often feel helpless and want someone else to solve my problems.
52. I am a very active person.
53. I have a lot of intellectual curiosity.
54. If I don't like people, I let them know it.
55. I never seem to be able to get organized.

56. At times I have been so ashamed I just wanted to hide.
57. I would rather go my own way than be a leader of others.
58. I often enjoy playing with theories or abstract ideas.
59. If necessary, I am willing to manipulate people to get what I want.
60. I strive for excellence in everything I do.

Enter your responses here—remember to enter responses *ACROSS* the rows.

SD = *Strongly Disagree*; D = *Disagree*; N = *Neutral*; A = *Agree*; SA = *Strongly Agree*

ENTER ACROSS

1 (SD)(D)(N)(A)(SA)	2 (SD)(D)(N)(A)(SA)	3 (SD)(D)(N)(A)(SA)	4 (SD)(D)(N)(A)(SA)	5 (SD)(D)(N)(A)(SA)
6 (SD)(D)(N)(A)(SA)	7 (SD)(D)(N)(A)(SA)	8 (SD)(D)(N)(A)(SA)	9 (SD)(D)(N)(A)(SA)	10 (SD)(D)(N)(A)(SA)
11 (SD)(D)(N)(A)(SA)	12 (SD)(D)(N)(A)(SA)	13 (SD)(D)(N)(A)(SA)	14 (SD)(D)(N)(A)(SA)	15 (SD)(D)(N)(A)(SA)
16 (SD)(D)(N)(A)(SA)	17 (SD)(D)(N)(A)(SA)	18 (SD)(D)(N)(A)(SA)	19 (SD)(D)(N)(A)(SA)	20 (SD)(D)(N)(A)(SA)
21 (SD)(D)(N)(A)(SA)	22 (SD)(D)(N)(A)(SA)	23 (SD)(D)(N)(A)(SA)	24 (SD)(D)(N)(A)(SA)	25 (SD)(D)(N)(A)(SA)
26 (SD)(D)(N)(A)(SA)	27 (SD)(D)(N)(A)(SA)	28 (SD)(D)(N)(A)(SA)	29 (SD)(D)(N)(A)(SA)	30 (SD)(D)(N)(A)(SA)
31 (SD)(D)(N)(A)(SA)	32 (SD)(D)(N)(A)(SA)	33 (SD)(D)(N)(A)(SA)	34 (SD)(D)(N)(A)(SA)	35 (SD)(D)(N)(A)(SA)
36 (SD)(D)(N)(A)(SA)	37 (SD)(D)(N)(A)(SA)	38 (SD)(D)(N)(A)(SA)	39 (SD)(D)(N)(A)(SA)	40 (SD)(D)(N)(A)(SA)
41 (SD)(D)(N)(A)(SA)	42 (SD)(D)(N)(A)(SA)	43 (SD)(D)(N)(A)(SA)	44 (SD)(D)(N)(A)(SA)	45 (SD)(D)(N)(A)(SA)
46 (SD)(D)(N)(A)(SA)	47 (SD)(D)(N)(A)(SA)	48 (SD)(D)(N)(A)(SA)	49 (SD)(D)(N)(A)(SA)	50 (SD)(D)(N)(A)(SA)
51 (SD)(D)(N)(A)(SA)	52 (SD)(D)(N)(A)(SA)	53 (SD)(D)(N)(A)(SA)	54 (SD)(D)(N)(A)(SA)	55 (SD)(D)(N)(A)(SA)
56 (SD)(D)(N)(A)(SA)	57 (SD)(D)(N)(A)(SA)	58 (SD)(D)(N)(A)(SA)	59 (SD)(D)(N)(A)(SA)	60 (SD)(D)(N)(A)(SA)

Now answer the three questions labeled A, B, and C below.

A. Have you responded to all of the statements? ______ Yes ______ No

B. Have you entered your responses across the rows? ______ Yes ______ No

C. Have you responded accurately and honestly? ______ Yes ______ No

ID#

Name ______________________ Age ______ Sex ______ Today's date ______

NEO Five-Factor Inventory-3 Profile
Form S (Adult)

Male

	T	N	E	O	A	C
Very High	≥75	≥37	≥43	≥43	≥44	≥47
	74	36	42			
	73		41	42	43	46
	72	35		41		
	71	34	40		42	45
	70	33		40		44
	69		39	39	41	
	68	32	38		40	43
	67	31		38		
	66		37		39	42
High	65	30		37		41
	64	29	36	36	38	
	63	28	35			40
	62			35	37	
	61	27	34	34	36	39
	60	26	33			38
	59			33	35	
	58	25	32			37
	57	24		32	34	
	56		31	31		36
Average	55	23	30		33	35
	54	22		30	32	
	53	21	29	29		34
	52				31	
	51	20	28	28		33
	50	19	27	27	30	32
	49					
	48	18	26	26	29	31
	47	17				
	46	16	25	25	28	30
	45		24	24	27	29
Low	44	15				
	43	14	23	23	26	28
	42			22		
	41	13	22		25	27
	40	12	21	21		26
	39	11			24	
	38		20	20	23	25
	37	10	19	19		
	36	9			22	24
	35		18	18		23
Very Low	34	8		17	21	
	33	7	17			22
	32	6	16	16	20	
	31				19	21
	30	5	15	15		20
	29	4		14	18	
	28		14			19
	27	3	13	13	17	
	26			12		18
	25	[illegible]	[illegible]	11	16	17

Female

	T	N	E	O	A	C
Very High	≥75	≥42	≥45	≥45	48	
	74	41	44	44		
	73	40	43		47	48
	72			43	46	47
	71	39	42			
	70	38		42	45	46
	69	37	41	41		45
	68		40		44	
	67	36		40		44
	66	35	39	39	43	43
High	65	34	38		42	
	64	33		38		42
	63		37		41	41
	62	32		37		
	61	31	36	36	40	40
	60	30	35			39
	59	29		35	39	
	58		34	34	38	38
	57	28				
	56	27	33	33	37	37
Average	55	26	32			36
	54	25		32	36	
	53		31	31		35
	52	24	30		35	34
	51	23		30	34	
	50	22	29	29		33
	49				33	32
	48	21	28	28		
	47	20	27		32	31
	46	19		27		30
	45	18	26	26	31	
Low	44		25		30	29
	43	17		25		28
	42	16	24		29	
	41	15		24		27
	40	14	23	23	28	26
	39		22			
	38	13		22	27	25
	37	12	21	21		
	36	11			26	24
	35	10	20	20	25	23
Very Low	34		19			
	33	9		19	24	22
	32	8	18	18		21
	31	7	17		23	
	30			17		20
	29	6	16	16	22	19
	28	5			21	
	27	4	15	15		18
	26	3	14		20	17
	≤25	[illegible]	13	14	19	16

Combined

	T	N	E	O	A	C
Very High	≥75	≥40	≥44	≥44	≥47	48
	74	39	43			
	73			43	46	47
	72	38	42	42	45	
	71	37	41			46
	70	36		41	44	45
	69		40			
	68	35		40	43	44
	67	34	39	39	42	43
	66	33	38			
High	65	32		38	41	42
	64		37	37		
	63	31	36		40	41
	62	30		36	39	40
	61	29	35			
	60			35	38	39
	59	28	34	34		38
	58	27	33		37	
	57	26		33	36	37
	56		32	32		36
Average	55	25	31		35	
	54	24		31		35
	53	23	30	30	34	
	52	22			33	34
	51		29	29		33
	50	21	28		32	
	49	20		28		32
	48	19	27	27	31	31
	47				30	
	46	18	26	26		30
	45	17	25	25	29	
Low	44	16				29
	43		24	24	28	28
	42	15	23		27	
	41	14		23		27
	40	13	22	22	26	26
	39	12				
	38		21	21	25	25
	37	11	20	20	24	24
	36	10				
	35	9	19	19	23	23
Very Low	34		18			
	33	8		18	22	22
	32	7	17	17	21	21
	31	6				
	30		16	16	20	20
	29	5	15	15		19
	28	4			19	
	27	[illegible]	14	14	18	18
	26			13		
	≤25	[illegible]	[illegible]	12	[illegible]	[illegible]

Your

NEO™ Summary

Paul T. Costa, Jr., PhD and Robert R. McCrae, PhD

The NEO Inventory measures five broad domains, or dimensions, of personality. Responses describing your thoughts, feelings, and goals can be compared with those describing others' to portray your personality.

This summary is intended to give you a general idea of what your personality is like. It is not a detailed report. If you completed the inventory again, or if someone else described you, you might score somewhat differently.

The NEO Inventory measures differences among people in general. It is not a test of intelligence or ability, and it is not intended to diagnose problems of mental health or adjustment. It does, however, give you some idea of what makes you unique in your ways of thinking, feeling, and interacting with others.

Compared with the responses of other people, your responses suggest that you can be described as:

☐ Sensitive, emotional, and prone to experience feelings that are upsetting.	☐ Generally calm and able to deal with stress, but you sometimes experience feelings of guilt, anger, or sadness.	☐ Secure, hardy, and generally relaxed, even under stressful conditions.
☐ Extraverted, outgoing, active, and high-spirited. You prefer to be around people most of the time.	☐ Moderate in activity and enthusiasm. You enjoy the company of others, but you also value privacy.	☐ Introverted, reserved, and serious. You prefer to be alone or with a few close friends.
☐ Open to new experiences. You have broad interests and are very imaginative.	☐ Practical, but willing to consider new ways of doing things. You seek a balance between the old and the new.	☐ Down-to-earth, practical, traditional, and pretty much set in your ways.
☐ Compassionate, good-natured, and eager to cooperate and avoid conflict.	☐ Generally warm, trusting, and agreeable, but you can sometimes be stubborn and competitive.	☐ Hardheaded, skeptical, proud, and competitive. You tend to express your anger directly.
☐ Conscientious and well-organized. You have high standards and always strive to achieve your goals.	☐ Dependable and moderately well-organized. You generally have clear goals but are able to set your work aside.	☐ Easygoing, not very well-organized, and sometimes careless. You prefer not to make plans.

PAR • 16204 N. Florida Ave. • Lutz, FL 33549 • 1.800.331.8378 • www.parinc.com

9 8 7 6 5 Reorder #RO-6799 Printed in the U.S.A.

Sum the COLUMNS to obtain raw scores for N, E, O, A, and C.
Plot raw scores on facing page to obtain *T* scores.

1 (4)(3)(2)(1)(0)	2 (0)(1)(2)(3)(4)	3 (0)(1)(2)(3)(4)	4 (0)(1)(2)(3)(4)	5 (0)(1)(2)(3)(4)
6 (0)(1)(2)(3)(4)	7 (0)(1)(2)(3)(4)	8 (0)(1)(2)(3)(4)	9 (4)(3)(2)(1)(0)	10 (0)(1)(2)(3)(4)
11 (0)(1)(2)(3)(4)	12 (4)(3)(2)(1)(0)	13 (0)(1)(2)(3)(4)	14 (4)(3)(2)(1)(0)	15 (4)(3)(2)(1)(0)
16 (4)(3)(2)(1)(0)	17 (0)(1)(2)(3)(4)	18 (4)(3)(2)(1)(0)	19 (4)(3)(2)(1)(0)	20 (0)(1)(2)(3)(4)
21 (0)(1)(2)(3)(4)	22 (0)(1)(2)(3)(4)	23 (4)(3)(2)(1)(0)	24 (4)(3)(2)(1)(0)	25 (0)(1)(2)(3)(4)
26 (0)(1)(2)(3)(4)	27 (4)(3)(2)(1)(0)	28 (4)(3)(2)(1)(0)	29 (0)(1)(2)(3)(4)	30 (4)(3)(2)(1)(0)
31 (4)(3)(2)(1)(0)	32 (0)(1)(2)(3)(4)	33 (4)(3)(2)(1)(0)	34 (0)(1)(2)(3)(4)	35 (0)(1)(2)(3)(4)
36 (0)(1)(2)(3)(4)	37 (0)(1)(2)(3)(4)	38 (0)(1)(2)(3)(4)	39 (4)(3)(2)(1)(0)	40 (0)(1)(2)(3)(4)
41 (0)(1)(2)(3)(4)	42 (4)(3)(2)(1)(0)	43 (0)(1)(2)(3)(4)	44 (4)(3)(2)(1)(0)	45 (4)(3)(2)(1)(0)
46 (4)(3)(2)(1)(0)	47 (0)(1)(2)(3)(4)	48 (4)(3)(2)(1)(0)	49 (0)(1)(2)(3)(4)	50 (0)(1)(2)(3)(4)
51 (0)(1)(2)(3)(4)	52 (0)(1)(2)(3)(4)	53 (0)(1)(2)(3)(4)	54 (4)(3)(2)(1)(0)	55 (4)(3)(2)(1)(0)
56 (0)(1)(2)(3)(4)	57 (4)(3)(2)(1)(0)	58 (0)(1)(2)(3)(4)	59 (4)(3)(2)(1)(0)	60 (0)(1)(2)(3)(4)

N = ______ E = ______ O = ______ A = ______ C = ______

A. Have you responded to all of the statements? Yes No

B. Do not score if this response is marked "No" Yes No

C. Do not score if this response is marked "No" Yes No

(CONFIDENTIAL गोपनीय)

SINHA ANXIETY SCALE

(SINHA W.A. SELF-ANALYSIS FORM)

Constructed and Standardized by

D. Sinha

Ex-Professor & Head of the Deptt. of Psychology
University of Allahabad
ALLAHABAD

निम्न सूचनाएँ परीक्षार्थी को स्वयं भरनी है

नाम .... उम्र .... वर्ष .... माह ....

विवाहित/अविवाहित । स्त्री/पुरुष

कक्षा .... स्कूल (या कालेज) ....

पिता (या अभिभावक) का व्यवसाय .... जाति ....

परिवार की संयुक्त मासिक आय ....

दिनांक ....

प्रकाशक

रूपा साइकोलॉजिकल सेन्टर

बी० १९/६० बी, डेवढ़ियाबीर, भेलूपुर, वाराणसी

निर्देश

अगले पृष्ठों पर आपकी सामाजिक और व्यवहारिक समस्याओं से सम्बन्धित कुछ वाक्य दिये हुए हैं । इन वाक्यों में उन्हीं बातों का उल्लेख है जो आप अपने दैनिक जीवन में अनुभव करते हैं और व्यवहार में लाते हैं.। इन वाक्यों का सम्बन्ध आपकी बुद्धि परीक्षा से नहीं बल्कि कुछ तथ्यों की जाँच से है ।

सूची में दी हुई प्रत्येक समस्या को ध्यान से पढ़िये । प्रत्येक समस्या के सामने **"हाँ"** या **"नहीं"** लिखा हुआ है । आपके व्यवहार व परिस्थिति में जो समस्या सत्य या असत्य हो उनमें से प्रत्येक के सामने "हाँ" या **"नही"** पर निशान (✓) लगाइये । जैसे :- "मुझे अपने ऊपर बिल्कुल विश्वास नहीं है" यदि यह वाक्य आपके व्यवहार में **सत्य** है तो **"हाँ"** के सामने निशान (✓) लगाइए और यदि असत्य है तो **"नही"** के सामने निशान लगाइए ।

सूची भरने के लिए आपको पूरी स्वतन्त्रता है । आपके उत्तर पूर्ण रूप से गोपनीय रखे जायेंगे । प्रत्येक समस्या को पढ़िए और उसके सामने अपने विचार के अनुसार निशान लगाइए ।

सभी समस्याओं पर निशान लगाना आवश्ध्यक है कृपया शीघ्रता से उत्तर दें ।

उत्तर शीघ्र दीजिए

प्रत्येक समस्या का उत्तर देना आवश्यक है।

क्रम संख्या		निशान (✓) लगाइये	
		हाँ	नहीं
१.	मुझे तेज सवारी पर चलने से घबराहट होती है।	हाँ	नहीं
२.	मै थोड़ी सी भी आवाज से घवड़ा जाता हूँ।	हाँ	नहीं
३.	विपरीत लिंग के व्यक्ति (Opposite sex) से मिलने पर मुझे कुछ घबराहट-सी मालूम होती है।	हाँ	नहीं
४.	घर के बाहर जाने पर कभी-कभी सन्देह होता है कि मैंने बक्स या दरवाजा बन्द किया या नहीं।	हाँ	नहीं
५.	मै अधिकतर यह सोचकर परेशान रहता हूँ कि कहीं लोग मेरा मजाक न उड़ाएँ।	हाँ	नहीं
६.	कभी-कभी मुझे सन्देह होता है कि मेरे मित्र गुप्त बातों को प्रकट न कर दें।	हाँ	नहीं
७.	प्रायः मुझमें अपराध की भावना होती है।	हाँ	नहीं
८.	कभी-कभी मैं नाखून कुतरता हूँ।	हाँ	नहीं
९.	मुझे प्रायः एक डर बना रहता है कि कहीं कोई आपित्त या दुर्भाय न टूट पड़े।	हाँ	नहीं
१०.	ठंडक के दिनों में भी मुझे बड़ी आसानी से पसीना आ जाता है।	हाँ	नहीं
११.	मुझे प्रायः बुरे और डरावने सपने दिखाई देते है।	हाँ	नहीं
१२.	मुझे कभी-कभी यह चिन्ता हो जाती है कि कहीं मैं नपुसंक न हो जाऊँ।	हाँ	नहीं
१३.	कभी-कभी इस विचार से मैं परेशान हो जाता हूँ कि अपने काम में अधिक प्रगति नहीं कर पाऊँगा।	हाँ	नहीं
१४.	अपनी आलोचना सुनकर मैं बहुत घबड़ा जाता हूँ	हाँ	नहीं
१५.	कभी-कभी अपने ऊपर इतनी आत्म-ग्लानि होती है कि मन करता है कि समाज से कहीं दूर भाग जाऊँ।	हाँ	नहीं

क्रम संख्या		निशान (✓) लगाइये	
१६.	यदि कोई मेरी गलतियाँ दूसरों के सामने कहता है तो मैं विचलित-सा हो जाता हूँ।	हाँ	नहीं
१७.	बीमारी के कीटाणुओं के भय से मैं शायद ही कभी घर के बाहर पानी पीता हूँ।	हाँ	नहीं
१८.	कभी-कभी मैं अकारण ही दुःखी हो जाता हूँ।	हाँ	नहीं
१९.	मुझे अधिकतर ऐसा लगता है कि दूसरे लोग मेरी उपेक्षा कर रहे हैं।	हाँ	नहीं
२०.	मैं बड़ी आसानी से धर्म-संकट में पड़ जाता हूँ।	हाँ	नहीं
२१.	किसी एक कार्य पर ध्यान केन्द्रित करना मेरे लिये प्रायः मुश्किल हो जाता है।	हाँ	नहीं
२२.	अक्सर मेरा जी मिचलाता है।	हाँ	नहीं
२३.	काम करते समय मेरे हाथ काँपते हैं।	हाँ	नहीं
२४.	मुझे कभी-कभी भय हो जाता है कि नये कपड़े पहन कर मैं बेढंगा न लगूँ।	हाँ	नहीं
२५.	मुझे यह जानकर परेशानी होती है कि मेरा मुँह शर्म से लाल होने जा रहा है।	हाँ	नहीं
२६.	मुझे अधिकतर ऐसा लगता है कि मेरा दिल जोर से धड़क रहा है।	हाँ	नहीं
२७.	मुझे दूसरों की अपेक्षा अधिक घबड़ाहट होती है।	हाँ	नहीं
२८.	मुझे अक्सर रोने की इच्छा होती है।	हाँ	नहीं
२९.	कभी-कभी चिन्ता के कारण मुझे नींद नहीं आती।	हाँ	नहीं
३०.	मुझे अपने से बड़े (निर्देशक, अध्यापक, अधीक्षक) से मिलने में परेशानी होती है।	हाँ	नहीं
३१.	कभी-कभी मैं बहुत बेचैन हो उठता हूँ।	हाँ	नहीं
३२.	दूसरों की गलतियों पर भी मैं शर्मिन्दा हो जाता हूँ।	हाँ	नहीं
३३.	जल्दी काम करने से मेरा दम फूलने लगता है।	हाँ	नहीं
३४.	मैं अपना काम काफी मानसिक तनाव की हालत में करता हूँ।	हाँ	नहीं

क्रम संख्या		निशान (✓) लगाइये	
३५.	अक्सर मुझे ऐसा लगता है कि मुझे कोई नहीं चाहता ।	हाँ	नहीं
३६.	मेरे सामने कठिन काम आने पर मैं काँपता हूँ या मुझे पसीना आने लगता है ।	हाँ	नही
३७.	कभी-कभी मैं सपने देखता हूँ कि बुरी तरह बीमार हो गया हूँ ।	हाँ	नहीं
३८.	कभी-कभी मैं ऐसे सपने देखता हूँ जो दूसरों से कहने लायक नहीं होते ।	हाँ	नहीं
३९.	किसी चीज के लिए प्रतीक्षा करना मेरे लिए एक परेशानी हो जाती है ।	हाँ	नहीं
४०.	मेरी भावनाओं को बड़ी जल्दी ठेस लग जाती है ।	हाँ	नहीं
४१.	मैं हमेशा किसी न किसी चीज के लिए परेशान रहता हूँ ।	हां	नहीं
४२.	मैं हरदम पेट की गड़बड़ी से परेशान रहता हूँ ।	हाँ	नही
४३.	किसी भी प्रकार के निश्चय पर पहुँचने में बहुत कठिनाई होती है ।	हाँ	नहीं
४४.	मैं कभी-कभी व्यर्थ की बातों के लिए भी चिन्तित हो जाता हूँ ।	हाँ	नहीं
४५.	मैं अधिकतर डरा करता हूँ कि कहीं मैं अपने मित्रों को न खो बैठूँ ।	हाँ	नहीं
४६.	कभी-कभी मैं इतना उत्तेजित हो जाता हूँ कि साफ-साफ बोल नहीं पाता ।	हाँ	नहीं
४७.	मुझे अन्य लोगों की अपेक्षा अधिक आत्म-संकोच (Self conscious) होता है ।	हाँ	नही
४८.	मुझे जीवन अधिकतर एक भार सा लगता है ।	हाँ	नहीं
४९.	मुझे अपने ऊपर बिलकुल विश्वास नही है ।	हाँ	नहीं
५०.	कभी-कभी मेरे लिए मानसिक स्थिरता बनाए रखना कठिन हो जाता है ।	हाँ	नहीं
५१.	जब बुरे सपने के कारण मेरी नींद टूट जाती है तो मेरे लिए फिर सोना मुश्किल हो जाता है ।	हाँ	नहीं
५२.	कभी-कभी मुझे छोटी-छोटी बातों पर भी लज्जा और क्षोभ होता है ।	हाँ	नहीं
५३.	जब मुझे किसी अनजान व्यक्ति से मिलना हो तो मुझे घबड़ाहट होती है ।	हाँ	नहीं
५४.	मेरी नीद रात में कई बार टूट जाती है ।	हाँ	नहीं
५५.	कभी-कभी मुझे ऐसा लगता है कि मैं समाज को मुँह दिखलाने लायक नहीं हूँ ।	हाँ	नहीं

क्रम संख्या		निशान (✓) लगाइये	
५६.	जब दो या अधिक लोग कानाफूसी करते हैं तो मुझे लगता है कि वे मेरे ही बारे में बात कर रहे है ।	हाँ	नहीं
५७.	यदि मुझसे कोई अनुचित सामाजिक व्यवहार हो जाता है तो मैं उसे भूल नहीं पाता ।	हाँ	नहीं
५८.	जीवन की बीती घटनाओं को सोचकर मुझे कुछ क्षोभ-सा होता है ।	हाँ	नहीं
५९.	कभी-कभी मैं यह सोचकर परेशान हो जाता हूँ कि बूढ़े होने पर मेरे बच्चे मेरा आदर नहीं करेंगे ।	हाँ	नहीं
६०.	यात्रा शुरू करने से पहले मैं कुछ चिन्तित हो जाता हूँ ।	हाँ	नहीं
६१.	मैं ऐसी परिस्थितियों में पड़ना पसन्द नहीं करता जिनमें निर्णय शीघ्र करना पड़ता है ।	हाँ	नहीं
६२.	मुझे अक्सर यह चिन्ता बनी रहती है कि मैं देखने में सुन्दर नहीं हूँ ।	हाँ	नहीं
६३.	कभी-कभी मुझे ऐसा लगता है कि मैं शीघ्र बूढ़ा होने लगा ।	हाँ	नहीं
६४.	यदि मुझे डाक्टर या सर्जन के पास दिखलाने के लिए जाना होता है तो मुझे घबड़ाहट होती है ।	हाँ	नहीं
६५.	कभी-कभी मुझे शंका हो जाती है कि मेरे मित्र मुझे धोखा न दें ।	हाँ	नहीं
६६.	जब मैं कोई नया काम करता हूँ तो मुझे परेशानी रहती है कि दूसरे समर्थन करेंगे या नहीं ।	हाँ	नहीं
६७.	मैं अपने स्वास्थ्य के विषय में अधिकतर चिन्तित रहा करता हूँ ।	हाँ	नहीं
६८.	लोगों के बीच भी मैं अधिकतर अकेला महसूस करता हूँ ।	हाँ	नहीं
६९.	जब मैं किसी व्यक्ति की प्रतीक्षा करता हूँ जिसने किसी निश्चित समय पर आने को कहा है तो मुझे अक्सर ऐसा लगता है कि शायद वह नहीं आयेगा ।	हाँ	नहीं
७०.	कभी-कभी मैं कुछ ऐसे कामों से परेशान हो जाता हूँ जिनको मैं स्पष्ट रूप से जानता नहीं ।	हाँ	नहीं
७१.	बहुत बार ऐसा होता है कि मैं साफ-साफ नहीं सोच सकता हूँ ।	हाँ	नहीं
७२.	बहुधा मैं यह निश्चित नहीं कर पाता हूँ कि किस तरह से काम करना मेरे लिए अच्छा होगा ।	हाँ	नहीं

क्रम संख्या		निशान (✓) लगाइये	
७३.	मैं बहुधा अपने बारे में अनिश्चित रहता हूँ ।	हाँ	नहीं
७४.	कभी-कभी मैं ऐसा सोच बैठता हूँ कि मैं किसी काम का नहीं हूँ ।	हाँ	नहीं
७५.	मुझे अधिकतर ऐसा लगता है कि यह संसार तथा मनुष्य दोनों की व्यर्थ है ।	हाँ	नहीं
७६.	असफल होने के भय से मुझे किसी काम को शुरू करने में हिचकिचाहिट होती है ।	हाँ	नहीं
७७.	सपनों में कभी-कभी मैं अपने निकट और प्रिय सम्बन्धियों की मृत्यु देखता हूँ ।	हाँ	नहीं
७८.	मैं शीघ्र ही थक जाता हूँ ।	हाँ	नहीं
७९.	मेरी हथेली में अक्सर पसीना आता है ।	हाँ	नहीं
८०.	इस डर से कि कहीं लोग मजाक न उड़ाएँ, मैं लोगों के सम्मुख बात-चीत करना पसन्द नही करता ।	हाँ	नही
८१.	मुझे अक्सर ऐसा लगता है कि मेरे ऊपर कोई आपत्ति आने वाली है ।	हाँ	नही
८२.	कभी-कभी मुझे ऐसा लगता है कि मुझे लोग पसन्द नहीं करते है ।	हाँ	नही
८३.	मैं अक्सर चिन्तित रहता हूँ कि मेरे भाग्य में क्या लिखा है ।	हाँ	नही
८४.	दूसरों के किए पर मुझे ही प्रायः दोषी ठहराया जाता है ।	हाँ	नहीं
८५.	मैं अक्सर छोटी-छोटी बातों के लिए भी परेशान रहता हूँ ।	हाँ	नहीं
८६.	मैं यह सोचकर कि शायद अपना वायदा पूरा न कर पाऊँ अक्सर परेशान हो जाता हूँ ।	हाँ	नहीं
८७.	कठिन परिस्थितियों में मैं बहुत उत्तेजित हो उठता हूँ ।	हाँ	नहीं
८८.	मुझे करीब-करीब हर समय भूख-सी लगती है ।	हाँ	नहीं
८९.	मैं अक्सर चिन्तित रहता हूँ कि भविष्य में शायद किसी संकट में न पड़ जाऊँ ।	हाँ	नहीं
९०.	यह चिन्ता मुझे परेशान करती है कि जब मैं बूढ़ा जो जाऊँगा तो मेरा स्वास्थ्य खराब न हो जाये ।	हाँ	नहीं
९१.	परिवार में दुर्घटना और मौत की संभावना सोचकर मैं परेशान हो जाता हूँ ।	हाँ	नहीं
९२.	मुझे इस बात की अक्सर चिन्ता रहती है कि अपने काम से निकाल न दिया जाऊँ ।	हाँ	नहीं
९३.	कभी-कभी मैं इतना उत्तेजित हो उठता हूँ कि मेरे लिए सोना कठिन हो जाता है ।	हाँ	नहीं

क्रम संख्या . निशान (✓) लगाइये

९४.	यह सोचकर मुझे चिन्ता हो जाती है कि एक दिन मैं भी बूढ़ा हो जाऊंगा ।	हाँ	नहीं
९५.	मैं अपनी बेचैनी शायद ही कभी छिपा पाता हूं ।	हाँ	नहीं
९६.	मैं विपरीत लिंग (Opposite sex) के लोगों से बात करते समय कुछ हकलाने-सा लगता हूँ ।	हाँ	नहीं
९७.	कभी मुझे ऐसा शक होने लगता है कि मेरे मित्र बूढ़े होने पर मेरी इज्जत नहीं करेंगे ।	हाँ	नहीं
९८.	बुढ़ापे से शारीरिक शक्ति के क्षीण होने की संभावना मुझे सताया करती है ।	हाँ	नहीं
९९.	कभी-कभी मैं यह सोचकर परेशान हो जाता हूं कि क्रोध में मैं किसी की हत्या न कर दूँ या भारी नुकसान न पहुँचा दूँ ।	हाँ	नहीं
१००.	इस बात की मुझे अधिकतर चिन्ता रहती है कि मेरे मरने के बाद मेरे परिवार की क्या दशा होगी ।	हाँ	नहीं

केवल परीक्षक के लिए

पृष्ठ	३	४	५	६	७	८	योग
अंक							

T. M. No. 458715

S. K. VERMA *(Chandigarh)*
N. N. WIG *(Chandigarh)*
D. PERSHAD *(Chandigarh)*

Consumable Booklet
of

P.G.I. H.Q. N-I

कृपया निम्न सूचनाएँ दीजिए–

नाम ______________________________

उम्र ______________ लिंग ______________

शिक्षा ______________________________

व्यवसाय ______________________________

निर्देश

आगे के पृष्ठों पर आपके शारीरिक व मानसिक स्वास्थ्य के बारे में कुछ प्रश्न लिखे हैं। इनको ध्यान से पढ़िये और जो बातें आपके बारे में अधिकतर ठीक हों उनके सामने वाले खाने में सही (√) का निशान बनाइये।

SCORING TABLE

AREA	A	B	Total Scores
SCORES	2	2	4

Estd. : 1971 ✆ (0562) 364926

NATIONAL PSYCHOLOGICAL CORPORATION

4/230, KACHERI GHAT, AGRA - 282 004 (U. P.) INDIA

AREA A

1. मैं जल्दी थक जाता हूँ। ☐

2. मैं अक्सर बीमार रहता हूँ। ☐

3. मैं सेहत के बारे में बहुत परेशान रहता हूँ। ☐

4. मुझे भूख कम लगती है। ☐

5. मुझे कब्ज़ की शिकायत रहती है। ☐

6. मुझे अक्सर सिर दर्द रहता है। ☐

7. मुझे सर्दी-जुकाम जल्दी हो जाता है। ☐

8. मुझे गला बार-बार साफ करना पड़ता है। ☐

9. मुझे चक्कर आते हैं। ☐

10. मुझे बार-बार पेशाब करने जाना पड़ता है। ☐

11. मुझे नींद देर से आती है या जल्दी टूट जाती है। ☐

12. मेरी साँस फूल जाती है। ☐

13. मेरा पेट अक्सर खराब रहता है। ☐

14. मेरा दिल जोर-जोर से धड़कने लगता है। ☐

15. मेरे शरीर में दर्द होता है। ☐

16. मेरे पेट से कीड़े निकले हैं। ☐

AREA B

17. मैं शर्मीले स्वभाव का हूँ। ☐
18. मैं बात का जल्दी बुरा मान जाता हूँ। ☐
19. मैं छोटी-छोटी बातों से घबड़ा जाता हूँ। ☐
20. मैं चिन्ता बहुत करता हूँ। ☐
21. मैं हर काम के लिये दूसरों की राय माँगता हूँ। ☐
22. मैं किसी बात का जल्दी फैसला नहीं कर पाता। ☐
23. मैं थोड़ी-सी नुक्ताचीनी (आलोचना) से बहुत परेशान हो जाता हूँ। ☐
24. अगर काम जल्दी करना हो तो मैं घबड़ा जाता हूँ। ☐
25. मैं जान-बूझकर धीरे-धीरे काम करता हूँ ताकि काम गलत न हो जाय। ☐
26. मैं नये लोगों से मिलने या नई जगह जाने से घबड़ा जाता हूँ। ☐
27. मैं अक्सर उदास रहता हूँ। ☑
28. मैं जल्दी रो पड़ता हूँ। ☐
29. मैं जल्दी निराश हो जाता हूँ। ☐
30. अगर जोर से आवाज़ हो तो मैं डर जाता हूँ। ☐
31. अचानक कोई सामने से आ जाये तो मैं घबड़ा जाता हूँ। ☐
32. किसी अफसर/बड़े आदमी के सामने मुझे पसीना आने लगता है। ☐
33. मेरा स्वभाव चिड़चिड़ा हो जाता है। ☑
34. मुझे गुस्सा जल्दी आजाता है। ☐
35. मुझे अँधेरे में डर लगता है। ☐
36. मुझे डरावने स्वप्न आते हैं। ☐
37. मुझे जिन्दगी बेकार (फिजूल) लगती है। ☐
38. मेरी जिन्दगी से तो मौत अच्छी है। ☐

DANCE MOVEMENT THERAPY SESSION

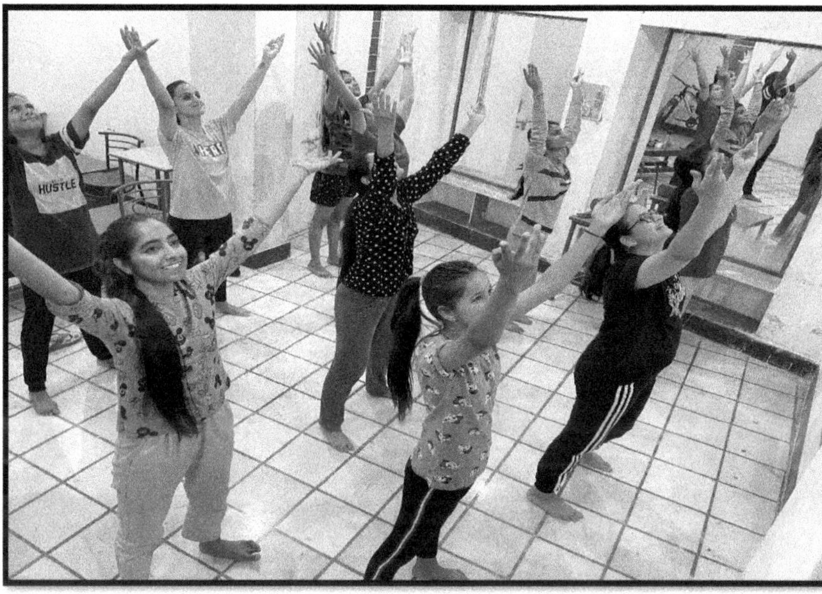

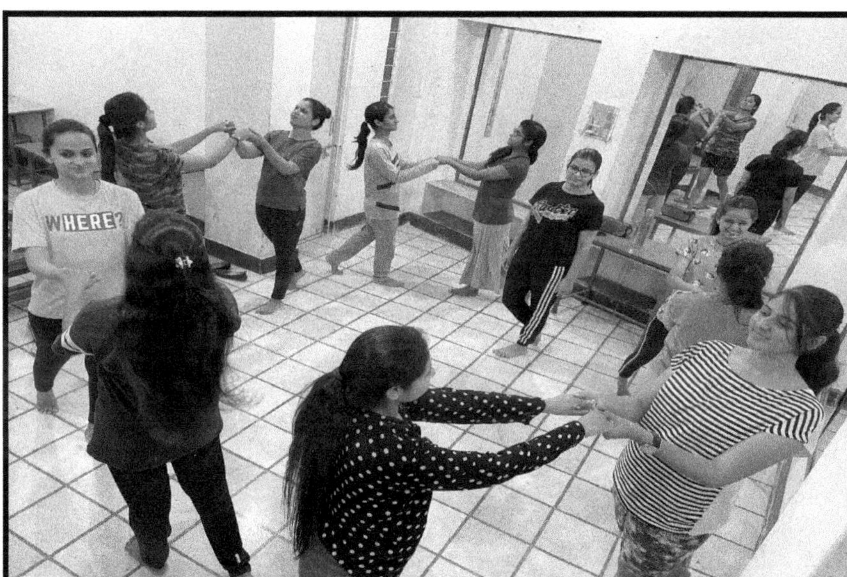

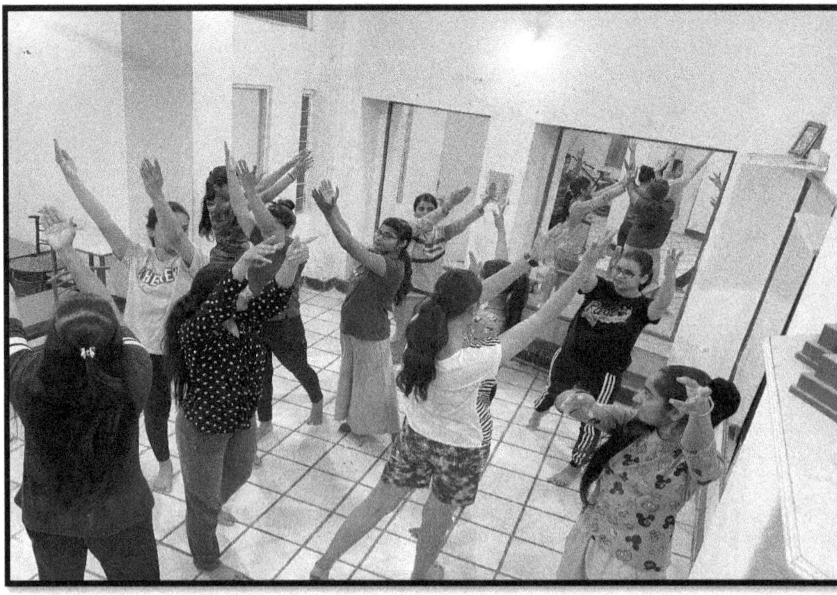

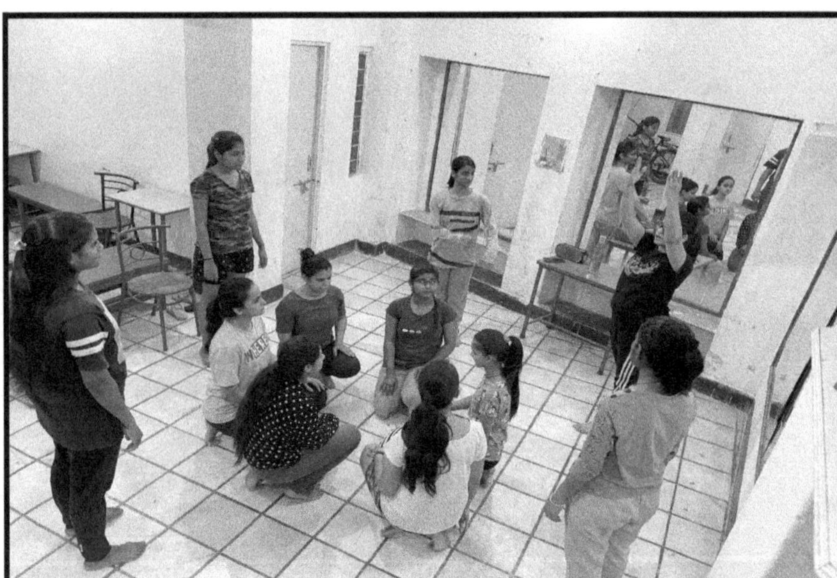

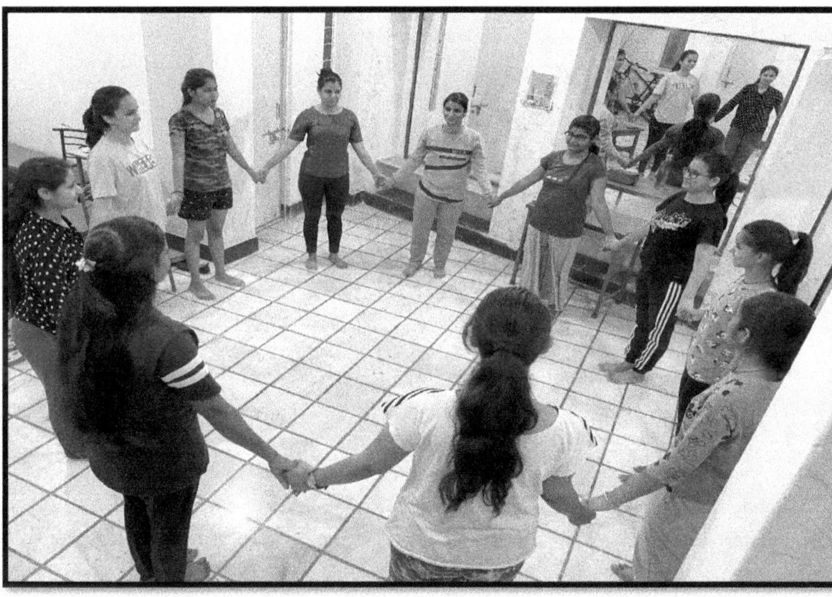

Effect of dance training on physical and mental health among adolescents

Authors

Ms Leni Nagda

Research Scholar

Department of Psychology

Mohanlal Sukhadia University

Udaipur, Rajasthan

&

Dr Tarun Kumar Sharma

Assistant Professor

Department of Psychology

Mohanlal Sukhadia University

Udaipur, Rajasthan

Abstract

The present research attempts to study the effect of Dance training on the physical and mental health among adolescents. The findings of the research would be helpful in understanding whether dance training has any potential positive effects on physical and mental health among adolescents. A sample of 120 adolescents was selected to study the effect of dance training and gender on physical and mental health among adolescents. The data was collected using PGI Health Questionnaire. The physical and mental health was better among those adolescents who were undergoing dance training in comparison to those who did not undergo any dance training. The female adolescents were found to have better physical and mental health than their male counterparts. The findings support the use of dance in the form of exercise for the overall well-being of individuals. The use of dance as a form of therapy is recommended for use by art therapists and dance-movement therapists.

Keywords: Dance, Physical health, Mental health, Dance-movement therapy

Dance has been considered a form of art which connects both body and mind and this conjunction is beneficial who indulge in this kind of art forms. Dance is not only an art of expression but is also a type of physical exercise which has positive impact on various aspects of an individual's development. Clinical Psychologists have been using various modes of art in the form of art therapy to heal and treat various mental health ailments. It is important to understand to what extent the dance training affects the emotional, cognitive, social development, an individual's temperament, attitude and overall well-being.

Indian philosophical though has emphasized on using dance and music for the benefit of an individual's spiritual, physical and mental well-being. India has various dance forms which are popular in different states of India. Katkak, Bharatnatyam, Kuchipudi are classical dance forms, whereas other forms of dance such as Punjab's Bhangra Rajasthan's Ghoomar, Gujarat's Garba and many other folk dance forms from tribal parts of India have also made worldwide recognition. The researches have been conducted with special reference to a particular dance form. Be it the rapid footwork of Kathak dancers which is useful in alleviating stress, anger and other emotional issues among the dancers.

Physical and Mental health

World Health Organisation (2019) defines "health as a state of complete physical, mental and social well-being and not merely the absence of disease or infirmity." Physical health is a state of physical well-being in which an individual is mechanically fit to perform their daily activities and duties without any problem.

Mohan (2017) explains the concept of health which is not the result of absent pathogens (viruses, bacteria) or the absence of psychological stress or conflicts, but the ability of the body to control those pathogenic factors sufficiently.

Physical health is an important part of individual's overall functioning and well-being. If an individual's physical health is affected, the other aspects such as social, intellectual, emotional, spiritual aspects are also affected. Some of the most obvious and serious signs that we are unhealthy appear physically. Assessment of physical health is vital to get an idea about overall well-being of an individual.

Another aspect of an individual is his/her mental health. It not only includes an individual's emotional well-being but it also related to how an individual is functioning in social setups. It is also determined by our cognitions, emotions, and overt actions. Mental health helps us in making connections with others, deciding our priorities in life, and to effectively function in our day-to-day lives. A person with sound mental health is able to face life challenges, his ability to deal with stress, life situations and relationships. Good mental health contributes to well-being of an individual. It instills positive traits such as self confidence, high self esteem and contributes to overall personality makeup of the individual.

Review of Previous Researches

The previous research work was studied to understand the background of the researches related to dance training. This review has also helped in framing research objectives and hypothesis in selecting appropriate variables for the study.

Dance movement therapy (DMT) is effective in controlling the level of depression among the patients who were suffering from mild to moderate level of depression. Koch et al (2019) found that DMT decreases depression and anxiety and increases quality of life and interpersonal and cognitive skills, whereas dance interventions increase psychomotor skills. Mastura & Haizan (2015) studied the effect of a 12-week low intensity dance exercise intervention in the treatment of hostility, anxiety and depression among overweight women which was found beneficial for their physical health and psychological well-being. Koch et al (2013) found that dance is effective for increasing quality of life and decreasing clinical symptoms such as depression and anxiety. Positive effects were also found on the increase of subjective well-being, positive mood, affect, and body image. Mohan, Singh & Dureja (2013) also explained the importance of physical health and its relationship with positive psychological traits such as optimism, health habits and locus of control. As the sportspersons are physically active and see life, people and events as good.

Iris B. (2012) found that dance improved the social relations/life. Kiepe et al (2012) found that ballroom dance improved balance and coordination in patients with Parkinson's disease and disease-specific quality of life in patients with heart failure. Dance movement therapy and ballroom dance seem beneficial for patients with breast cancer, depression, Parkinson's disease, diabetes and heart failure. It has been found that Dance movement Therapy can create a good environment for cognitive development. It is beneficial for the most number of children and implementable for maximum number of teachers.

Jeong et al (2005) suggested that DMT may stabilize the sympathetic nervous system. DMT may be effective in beneficially modulating concentrations of serotonin and dopamine, and in improving psychological distress in adolescents with mild depression. Gronlund, Renck & Weibull (2005) found that a minimum of ten weeks of dance movement therapy improved the motor function and also reduced the behavioural and emotional symptoms of boys aged 5–7 diagnosed with ADHD. Leventhal & Chang (1991) concluded that dance movement therapy can make to the treatment of battered women. By motivating female victims of domestic violence to act, dance movement therapy addresses patterns of helplessness, ambivalence, and inactivity. Dance movement interventions help women internalize a positive self-concept as well as gain physical and emotional control.

Crain, McLaughlin & Eisenhart (1983) studied that Educable Mentally Retarded (EMR) adolescents may exhibit problems in social and physical development in comparison with their normal peers. The purpose of this investigation was to study the effects of a 10 week dance program on EMR adolescents. It was found that nature of participation, consistency of participation, and the design of the curriculum affect the improvement of social and physical behaviours such as cooperation, dance skills, increased movement repertoire, rhythms, leadership and successful peer teaching.

In the above review of previous researches, it has been found that dance and dance movement therapy has been used for benefit and treatment of patients suffering from depression, attention deficit hyperactivity disorder, Parkinson's disease, breast cancer, mental retardation etc. Dance also has been found to improve the quality of life, social relationships and mood among the users. Looking at the number of adolescents who are undergoing dance training at various dance training centres, it becomes important to study whether these positive effects of dance training are visible among them as well or not. Lack of empirical data on dance training and its effect on an individual's physical and mental health has led us to formulate the following research objectives.

Objectives

The following research objectives and hypotheses have been framed:

To study the effect of dance training on physical health among adolescents

To study the effect of gender on physical health among adolescents

To study the effect of dance training on mental health among adolescents

To study the effect of gender on mental health among adolescents

Hypotheses:

H0: There is no difference between the physical health of Dance Trainee and Non Dance Trainee.

H0: There is no difference between mental health of Dance Trainee and Non Dance Trainee.

H0: There is no difference between the physical health of Males and Females.

H0: There is no difference between mental health of Males and Females.

Method

Sample:

The sample comprised of 120 adolescents selected in two groups. Each group consisted of 60 adolescents including 30 males and 30 females. In the first group, 60 adolescents who were taking dance training were included. In the second group 60 adolescents who were not receiving any type of dance training were included. First group is mentioned as 'Dance trainees' (DT) and the second group is mentioned as 'Non dance trainees' (NDT) in this research. Purposive method of sampling was used for selecting the sample. The sample of the first group was selected from different dance Institutes which were operational in Udaipur district of Rajasthan. A list was created by including male and female adolescents who were receiving dance training in these institutes and were in the age group of 18-30 years. The sample of second group was selected from schools and colleges. The data collection was done during the between October to December 2019.

Inclusion criteria: Those adolescents who were in the age bracket of 18-30 years and had undergone at least last 3 months of dance training were considered for inclusion in the dance trainee group. The age bracket was kept same for 'non dance trainees' group as well.

Variables:

Independent Variables:

a. Dance Training : Dance Trainee, No Dance Trainee

b. Gender : Male, Female

Dependent Variable:

a. Psychophysical Health (Physical health and Mental health) – Psychophysical health was measured by using PGI Health Questionnaire by S.K. Verma (1971). This questionnaire's Part-A measures Physical health whereas Part-B measures Mental health.

Result and Discussion

After the data collection and data entry were over, the obtained data was analyzed by using Statistical Package for Social Scientists (SPSS). The data was analyzed by using Analysis of Variance technique..

Dance Training and Health

Physical health

From Table 2, it is evident that the physical health is better among the adolescents who had been receiving dance training in comparison to those who were not receiving dance training. In the score obtained by PGI Health Questionnaire, the lesser are the score, the better is the health is. There was a significant effect of dance training on physical health at $t\,(1{,}118) = -16.061$, $p < .000$, there was significantly lower mean score of physical health among dance trainees ($M = 1.15$, $SD = 1.27$) than the non-dance trainees ($M = 6.38$, $SD = 2.17$).

Table 2 : Mean, S.D. and t-values : Dance Training and Health

		N	Mean	SD	Std. Error	t	df	p-value
Physical Health	Dance Trainee	60	1.15	1.273	.164	-16.061	118	.000
	Non Dance Trainee	60	6.38	2.179	.281			
Mental Health	Dance Trainee	60	1.20	1.054	.136	-14.065	118	.000
	Non Dance Trainee	60	8.03	3.612	.466			

Mental health

Similarly, the mental health is also better among the adolescents who had been receiving dance training in comparison to those who were not receiving dance training. There was a significant effect of dance training on mental health at t (1,118) = -14.065, $p < .000$, there was significantly lower mean score of mental health among dance trainees (M = 1.20, SD = 1.05) than the non-dance trainees (M = 8.03, SD = 3.61).

Gender and Health

Physical health

From Table 2, it is evident that the physical health is better among the female adolescents than male adolescents. There was a significant effect of gender on mental health at t (1,118) = 2.345, $p < .021$, there was significantly lower mean score of physical health among female adolescents (M = 4.43, SD = 3.60) than the male adolescents (M = 3.10, SD = 2.52).

Mental health

Similarly, the mental health is also better among the female adolescents than male adolescents. There was a significant effect of gender on mental health at t (1,118) = 3.334, $p < .001$, there was significantly lower mean score of mental health among female adolescents (M = 3.35, SD = 2.67) than the male adolescents (M = 5.88, SD = 5.244)

Table 3: Mean, S.D. and t-values: Gender and Health

		N	Mean	Std. Deviation	Std. Error	t	df	p-value
Physical health	Male	60	4.43	3.605	.465	2.345	118	.021
	Female	60	3.10	2.529	.327			
Mental health	Male	60	5.88	5.244	.677	3.334	118	.001
	Female	60	3.35	2.673	.345			

The findings obtained suggest that dance training has positive effect on both physical health and mental health among the adolescents. It is concluded that those adolescents who undergo dance training have better physical and mental health than the adolescents who do not undergo any kind of dance training. Gender has also found to have significant effect on physical health and mental health. Female adolescents have better physical and mental health than male adolescents.

Dance training provides the dancers a sense of control on their physical movements and their body which instill confidence among them. Regular dance practice makes the dancer's body soft and flexible which results in various physical health-related benefits. It also provide peace of mind as the dancers have to concentrate on their body movements, they need to connect their thought processes with the body movements. These kinds of exercises prove to be helpful for both physical health of dancers and mental capabilities such as confidence, perseverance, organization, dogged pursuit etc. The physical processes involved in dance such as the ability to balance the body, maintaining postures and gestures, the ability to express or communicate through non-verbal signs, the ability to control muscles, constricting and relating the muscles exert such powerful impact on the individual's overall personality and health.

Dance provides the dancers to connect to their inner world, their emotions which work for liberation and growth of an individual. It also develops sense of self worth; improve an individual's self concept and self esteem. Various dance forms are also a part of aerobic exercises. Aerobic exercises have proven benefits on cardiac illnesses, stress and related diseases, chronic pain, obesity and other physical health related illnesses.

Dance Movement therapy is also used for treatment of mental disorders. The American Dance Therapy Association defines dance movement therapy as the psychotherapeutic use of movement to further the emotional, cognitive, physical and social integration of the individual. The use of dance in the form of dance movement therapy is helpful for those individual who have social, psychological, physical impairments. This therapy is provided in individual settings; where one person is provided such therapy, in couples setting; where both the partners participate in the therapeutic process; or in family settings as well.

The cases of various forms of dementia are on the rise. The dance training has been found to be effective in counteracting the age-related cognitive decline. The researchers have recommended social dancing as an important tool for healthy ageing and living. Social dancing also improved the psychological make-up of an individual as the earlier isolated person gets involved with other in the group as a result of which the social life is also improved. The feeling of connectedness with others in the society also provide positive atmosphere.

Conclusion

Dance training is a type of physical activity which helps in alleviating physical and mental health related issues. As health is a dynamic processes and individuals have to put efforts for healthy life and overall-well being. Dance training is one of such ways by which one can overcome physical and mental health challenges.

References

Barton, E. J. (2011). Movement and mindfulness: a formative evaluation of dance/ movement and yoga therapy program with participants experiencing severe mental illness. American Journal of Dance Therapy, Vol 33, Issue 2, Page No. 157-181

Behrends, A. and Muller, S. and Dziobek, I. (2012). Moving in and out of synchrony : A concept for a new intervention fostering empathy through interactional movement and dance. Vol 39, Issue 2, Page No. 107-116. Retrieved from http://scholar.cnki.net/detail/sjestemp_U/SJ

Brauninger, I. (2012). The efficiency of dance movement therapy group on improvement of quality of life : A randomized control trial. Vol 39, Issue 4, Page No. 293-303. Retrieved from www.journals.elsevier.com

Brooklyn, L. Exploring dance/movement therapy to treat women with posttraumatic stress disorder. Retrieved fromhttp://www1.uwindsor.ca/criticalsocialwork/dancemovementtherapy

Chatterjee, A. (2013).The Therapeutic Value of Indian Classical, Folk and Innovative Dance Forms. Rupkatha Journal on Interdisciplinary Studies in Humanities Vol. V, No. 1, 2013. Retrieved from http://rupkatha.com/the-therapeutic-value-of-indian-classical-folk-and-innovative-dance-forms/

Colucci, J.Dance Therapy and Relaxation Therapy: Effects on Anxiety. Saint Anselm College, Dept. of Psychology. Retrieved from http://www.anselm.edu/internet/psych/theses/seniors2002/colucci/#abstract

Corteville, M. K. (2009). Dance Your Way to Communication: Dance Movement Therapy to Increase Self-Esteem, Poor Body Image, and Communication Skills in High School Females. Student Counselling& Personal Services Commons. Retrieved from http://digitalcommons.brockport.edu/edc_theses/21/

Crain, C.& McLoughlin, J.& Eisenhart, M. (1983). The Social and Physical Effects of a 10-Week Dance Program on Educable Mentally Retarded Adolescents. Education and Training of the Mentally Retarded. Retrieved from http://www.jstor.org/stable/23877241?seq=1#page_scan_tab_contents

Dr. Rainbow, H.T. H. (2014). Effects of dance/movement therapy on the disease symptoms in breast cancer patients undergoing radiotherapy. The HKU Scholars Hub. Retrieved from http://hub.hku.hk/handle/10722/197779

Gammo M. E. (2009). Dance as Therapy for Individuals with Parkinson Disease. Retrieved from www.ncbi.nlm.nih.gov/pmc/articles/pmc2780534

Gronlund, E. and Renck, B. and Weibull, J. (2005). Dance/Movement Therapy as an Alternative Treatment for Young Boys Diagnosed as ADHD: A Pilot Study, American Journal of Dance therapy, Vol 27, Issue 2, Page No. 63-85. Retrieved from http://www.researchgate.net/publication/227238006_DanceMovement_Therapy_as_an_Alternative_Treatment_for_Young_Boys_Diagnosed_as_ADHD_A_Pilot_Study

Jeong, Y. J.A. and Hong, S. C. and Lee, M. S.& Park, M. and Kim, Y. K.& Suh, C.M. (2005). Dance Movement Therapy improves emotional responses and modulates neurohormones in adolescents with mild depression, International Journal of Neuroscience, Vol 115, Issue 12. Retrieved from http://www.tandfonline.com/doi/abs/10.1080/00207450590958574#.Vfv0jNKqqko

Jojhar, M.& Shah M.& Taha (2015). Effect of Low Intensity Dance Exercise: Hostility, Anxiety and Depression among Sedentary Overweight Women in Malaysia, Universal Journal of Psychology Vol. 3(3), Dept. of Social Science, University of Tenaga National, Malaysia. Retrieved from http://www.hrpub.org/journals/article_info.php?aid=2512

Karpati, F. J. & Giacosa, C.& Foster, N. E.V. & Virginia B & Penhune & Hyde, Krista L. Annals of the New York Academy of Sciences Volume 1337Dance and the brain: a review (2015). Retrieved from http://onlinelibrary.wiley.com/doi/101111/nyas.12632/abstract

Sophie M.& Stockigt & Keil, T. (2012). Effects of dance therapy and ballroom dances on physical and mental illnesses: A systematic review, Vol 39, Issue 5, Page No. 404- 411. Retrieved from http://www.sciencedirect.com/science/article/pii/ S0197455612000998

Koch, S. C., Wirtz, G., Harter, C., Weisbrod, M., Winkler, F., Pröger, A., et al. (2019). Embodied self in trauma and self-harm: effects of flamenco therapy on traumatized in-patients. *A pilot study. J. Loss Trauma* 24, 441–459. doi: 10.1080/15325024.2018.1507472

Koch, S.& Kunj, T.& Lykou, S.& Cruz, R. (2014). The joy dance Specific effects of a single dance intervention on psychiatric patients with depression, Vol. 41 Issue 1. Retrieved from http://www.adta.org/Resources/Documents/Koch%20-%20The%20joy%20dance%20study.pdf

Koch, S.& Kunj, T.& Lykou, S.& Cruz, R. (2013). Effects of Dance Movement Therapy and Dance on Health-Related Psychological Outcomes: A Meta-Analysis. The Arts in Psychotherapy. 41. 10.1016/j.aip.2013.10.004.

Leventhal, F., & Chang, M. (1991). Dance/movement therapy with battered women: A paradigm of action. *American Journal of Dance Therapy*, *13*(2), 131–145. https://doi.org/10.1007/bf00844142

Mastura, J. & Shah, M. & Haizan, T. (2015). Effect of Low Intensity Dance Exercise: Hostility, Anxiety and Depression among Sedentary Overweight Women in Malaysia. Universal Journal of Psychology. 3. 73-79. 10.13189/ujp.2015.030303.

Mohan, J. (2017, March 23). *Seminar on "Positive Psychology and Spirituality for Holistic Health" at Amity*. India Education,Education News India,Education News | India Education Diary. https://indiaeducationdiary.in/seminar-positive-psychology-spirituality holistic-health-amity/

Mohan, J., Singh, K., & Dureja, G. (2013). Optimism, Health Habits and Locus of Control between Sportspersons and Non-Sportspersons. *International Journal of Sports Science and Engineering*, *07*(01), 26–030. http://www.worldacademicunion.com/journal/SSCI/SSCIvol07no01paper05.pdf

Sanderson, P. (2008). The arts, social inclusion and social class: The case of dance, British Educational Research Journal, Vol 34, No. 4. Retrieved from http://onlinelibrary.wiley.com/doi/10.1080/01411920701609349/abstract

World Health Organisation. (2019). *Constitution*. Who.Int. https://www.who.int/about/who-we-are/constitution

COMPARISON OF THE LEVEL OF ANXIETY AMONG DANCERS AND NON-DANCERS*

BY

MS LENI NAGDA♣

Research Scholar, Department of Psychology, Mohanlal Sukhadia University, Udaipur, Rajasthan

lenibhatt@gmail.com

DR TARUN KUMAR SHARMA

Assistant Professor, Department of Psychology
Mohanlal Sukhadia University, Udaipur, Rajasthan

tarun.udpr@gmail.com

ABSTRACT

Dance training requires an individual to engage in the dance physically, mentally, cognitively and emotionally. Various sources have revealed that every one in five persons in the 15-29 age groups suffer from anxiety, depression or some other kind of psycho-neurotic symptoms. It is important to understand whether dance training has any effect on the level of anxiety among adolescents. A sample of 120 adolescents was selected to study the effect of dance training and gender on the level of anxiety. The data was collected using Sinha Anxiety Scale. The effect of dance training on anxiety was found significant. The main effect of gender and the interaction effect of gender and dance training on the level of anxiety were not found to be significant. The findings support the use of dance based therapies such as dance-movement therapy for enhancing well-being.

KEYWORDS

Dance, Dance-movement therapy, Anxiety, Dance training.

INTRODUCTION

* Received 05 Jan 2021, Accepted 18 Jan 2021, Published 20 Feb 2021

♣ Correspondence Author

People need to be physically active to improve their overall health and fitness and prevent diseases. Physical activity means any movement of the body which involves using muscles and expands energy. Various researches in the past have shown that a total of two and a half hour physical activity per week like brisk walking, playing basketball, swimming, running, cycling and dancing reduces the risk of many chronic diseases. Research shows that doing exercise influences the release and uptake of feel-good chemicals called endorphins in the brain. Dance training requires an individual to engage in the dance physically, mentally, cognitively and emotionally.

Dance is a physical activity which involves a series of movements matching the speed and rhythm of music. Dance is a rhythmic activity, which is performed either in groups or individually. Dance can be one of the fun ways by which people particularly children and adolescents can incorporate movement and fitness in their routines. Dancing is an activity through which dancers learn to coordinate muscles to move through proper positions.

Indian philosophical though has emphasized on using dance and music for the benefit of an individual's spiritual, physical and mental well-being. India has various dance forms which are popular in different states of India. Katkak, Bharatnatyam, Kuchipudi are classical dance forms, whereas other forms of dance such as Punjab's Bhangra Rajasthan's Ghoomar, Gujarat's Garba and many other folk dance forms from tribal parts of India have also made worldwide recognition.

Dance has proven benefits on the physical health, but health not only includes the physical health aspects. World Health Organization (2019) defines "health as a state of complete physical, mental and social well-being and not merely the absence of disease or infirmity."

Review of Previous Researches

The previous research work was studied to understand the background of the researches related to dance training. This review has also helped in framing research objectives and hypothesis in selecting appropriate variables for the study.

Karkou, Aithal, Zubala and Meekums (2019) conducted a systematic review of studies that aimed to explore the effectiveness in the use of dance movement therapy with people with depression. Qualitative findings suggest there was a decrease in depression scores in favor of DMT groups. Groenlund, Renck, and Vaboe (2006) have found that depression in teenage girls was alleviated by three months of dance/movement therapy.

Mastura, Mardian and Haizan (2015) studied the effect of a 12-week low intensity dance exercise intervention in the treatment of hostility subscale, anxiety subscale and depression subscale among overweight women working in Malaysia in an attempt of Sports for all. It is concluded that low intensity dance therapy exercise intervention of "Aero mass" had contributed greatly to the positive findings concerning physical health and psychological well-being among overweight women in Malaysia.

DeMesa-Simpson (2014) studied the relationship between dance movement classes and disruptive behaviour was analyzed in a sample of 45 at risk students in an urban high school setting. The findings supported the hypothesis that a) dance classes can be utilized as an intervention to reduce stress and b) students who participate in dance programs in public school settings will develop self-control, self-regulation and exhibit less disruptive behaviour.

Sabine K., Teresa K., Sissy L. & Robyn C. (2014) evaluated the effectiveness of dance movement therapy (DMT) and the therapeutic use of dance for the treatment of health-related psychological problems. Results suggested that DMT and dance are effective for increasing quality of life and decreasing clinical symptoms such as depression and anxiety. Positive effects were also found on the increase of subjective well-being, positive mood, affect, and body image.

Mohan (2009) emphasized the role of sports and life style related factors in promoting well-being and excellence among those who are involved in various forms of sports. Similar to the sports, dance training also involves physical activity; it fosters various neurotransmitters which are helpful for positive healthy life. Jeong et al. (2005) found that dance movement therapy helps in stabilizing the sympathetic nervous system. DMT also improves the level of serotonin and dopamine, which is helpful in alleviating mild to moderate level of depression.

Various studies have been conducted on psychological and physical factors of dance movement therapy like effect of DMT on Depression, Cancer, Dementia, Autism but only few empirical studies are available on factors like health, personality of dance trainee, effect of DMT on anxiety in India.

Objectives

The following research objectives and hypotheses have been framed:

- To study the difference in the level of anxiety among dancers and non-dancers adolescents
- To study the difference in the level of anxiety among male and female adolescents
- To study the interaction effect of dance training and gender on level of anxiety among adolescents

Hypotheses:

- H0: There is no difference between the level of anxiety between dancers and non-dancers adolescents
- H0: There is no difference between the level of anxiety between male and female adolescents
- H0: There is no interaction effect of dance training and gender on the level of anxiety

Method

Sample:

The sample comprised of 120 adolescents selected in two groups. Each group consisted of 60 adolescents including 30 males and 30 females. In the first group, 60 adolescents who were taking dance training were included. In the second group 60 adolescents who were not receiving any type of dance training were included. Purposive method of sampling was used for selecting the sample. The sample of the first group was selected from different dance Institutes which were operational in Udaipur district of Rajasthan. A list was created by including male and female adolescents who were receiving dance training in these institutes. The sample of second group was selected from schools and colleges. The data collection was done between October to December 2019.

Inclusion criteria: Those adolescents who had received at least 3 months of dance training were considered for inclusion in the dance trainee group. This training should be received in the last three months. Prior training with any gap was not considered.

Variables:

Independent Variables:

a. Dance Training :
    - Dancers
    - Non-dancers

b. Gender :
    - Male adolescents
    - Female adolescents

Dependent Variable:

a. Anxiety – The level of Anxiety was measured by using Sinha Anxiety Scale by D. N. Sinha (1976).

Result

After the data collection and data entry were over, the obtained data was analyzed by using Statistical Package for Social Scientists (SPSS). The results were analyzed by using Mean, S.D. and t-values.

- For Sinha Anxiety Scale, the highest the score, the more is the level of anxiety. Among the four groups, the level of anxiety is highest for female adolescents who are not receiving any dance training. The level of anxiety is lowest for male adolescents who are receiving dance training.
- The mean anxiety score for adolescents who are not receiving any dance training is higher than those adolescents who are receiving dance training.
- The mean anxiety score for female adolescents is higher than male adolescents

Table 1: Mean and Standard Deviation of Anxiety

Gender	Trainee	Mean	Standard Deviation	N
Male	Non-Dance	25.7	7.40	30
	Dance	22.73	5.80	30
	Total	24.21	6.76	60
Female	Non-Dance	28.53	9.09	30

	Dance	22.5	4.89	30
	Total	25.51	7.85	60
Total	Non-Dance	27.11	8.34	60
	Dance	22.61	5.32	60
	Total	20.27	8.08	120

The main effect of dance training on anxiety was found significant at .01 levels. The adolescents who were undergoing dance training, experienced less anxiety as compared to those who were not taking any dance training. There was a significant effect of dance training on anxiety at F= 12.44, p< .000, there was significantly higher mean score of anxiety for non-dance trainee adolescents (M= 27.11, SD 8.34) than the mean score of dance trainee adolescents (M= 22.61, SD= 5.32). The result concluded that dance training has significant effect on the level of anxiety level among adolescents.

The main effect of gender on anxiety was not found significant. Similarly, the interaction effect of dance training and gender was also not found significant.

Table 4.2 Analysis of Variance

Source of Variation	*Sum of Square*	*df*	*Mean Square*	*F*	*P-value*
Gender	50.7	1	50.7	1.038	0.310
Dance training	607.5	1	607.5	12.44	0.000*
Gender * Dance training	70.53	1	70.53	1.444	0.232
Within Groups	5663.13	116	40.02		
Total	6391.86	119			

* Statistically significant at .001 levels

Discussion

Dance training involves an individual to involve physically, mentally, emotionally and cognitively in this art form. Dance training has proven benefits on the physical health as it provides flexibility to the body, it also lessens body pain associated with various diseases, it also improves cardiac and pulmonary health of individuals. Dancing also works as an energy booster activity. As dancing involves a lot of physical activity, it improves aerobic power of lungs thereby providing more oxygen to blood which alleviates many physical health related issues. A sound physical health is also supportive for a sound mental health.

Dance training is also helpful in controlling level of depression, anxiety and related mental health ailments. Dance training requires an individual to be a part of social groups as they join and become a part of a dance class group. It provides opportunities for social interaction, especially with the same age groups in a digital age scenario where most of the time, people are seen occupied with their mobile phones or other electronic devices. A feeling of shared common goal of learning dance also strengthens the interpersonal relationships and bonding among the dance trainees, which is one of the important factors in promoting well-being.

Dancing involves using on some form of music. This activity itself is enjoyable in nature and leads to improvement in mood which thereby reduces the level of stress, anxiety and depression among the dance trainees. As dance is accompanies by listening to some form of music which activates certain brain areas, whereas on the other hand, dancing improves body flexibility and balance by activating sensory and motor neural circuits. Dancing has been found to be helpful in increasing the level of certain neurotransmitters which are considered as mood-improving chemicals. It has been found that dancing helps in the release of dopamine which is a feel-good hormone.

Dancing provides a sense of touch where individuals form one-to-one physical contact in the form of touch, this also improves the mood and provides happiness among those involved. When the dancers perform their art form in front of the peer group or at any other family or other platform, it boosts the level of self confidence among the learners which also reduces anxiety and provides happiness. This way, dance is also helpful in controlling social anxiety related issues.

Through dancing, people express their emotions, by using various body gestures, postures and facial expressions. It is one of the ways of catharsis and leads to more emotional control, emotional balance and emotional regulation and stability among the learners.

Conclusion

The findings obtained suggest that dance training has positive effect in controlling the level of anxiety among the adolescents. It is concluded that those adolescents who undergo dance training experience less anxiety than the adolescents who do not undergo any kind of dance training. Gender differences in the level of anxiety among the adolescents have not been found significant. The psychotherapeutic use of dance based therapies need to be emphasized.

References

DeMesa-Simpson D.The impact of dance/movement classes on adolescent behavior in an urban high school setting (2014). Theses and Dissertations. 435. https://rdw.rowan.edu/etd/435

Groenlund, E., Renck, B., & Vaboe, N. G. (2006). How depressed teenage girls can be helped by dance movement therapy. In Presentation on the 2nd International Research Colloquium in Dance Therapy, Feb. 10–11, 2006.

Hariharan, M & Gadiraju, P & Rana, S. (2014). Biopsychosocial Approach to Health Care: Towards Optimizing the Outcome, pp 205-219. Narendra Publishing House. ISBN: 978-93-82471-82-0..

Jeong, Y. J., Hong, S. C., Lee, M., Park, M. C., Kim, Y. K., & Suh, C. M. (2005). Dance/movement therapy improves emotional responses and modulates neurohormones in adolescents with mild depression. International Journal of Neuroscience, 115(12), 1711–1720.

Karkou, V., Aithal, S., Zubala, A., & Meekums, B. (2019). Effectiveness of Dance Movement Therapy in the Treatment of Adults With Depression: A Systematic Review With Meta-Analyses. *Frontiers in psychology*, *10*, 936. https://doi.org/10.3389/fpsyg.2019.00936

Mastura J , Mardian S , Haizan T (2015). Effect of Low Intensity Dance Exercise: Hostility, Anxiety and Depression among Sedentary Overweight Women in Malaysia. Universal Journal of Psychology, 3(3), 73 - 79.

Mohan, J.(2009) Recent Advances in Sports Psychology. Friends Publication, Delhi, India

World Health Organisation. (2019). *Constitution.* Who.Int. https://www.who.int/about/who-we-are/constitution

CHAPTER 2

REVIEW OF LITERATURE

A literature review provides an explanation, summary and assessment of any particular area of research or theory by examining the content available in various journals, books, web resources, e-journals and other research articles from other relatable sources. Review of Literature is important in giving us an understanding about the research trends and research gap on a particular topic. While exploring a particular topic and to express to the readers how a research fits within a greater field of study the literature reviews are an important part of the research which not only provides an overview of the chosen topic but also provides important insights to the research so as to carefully plan the research, its objectives, methodology, tools etc.

2.1 Importance of Review of Literature

Any subject or area of research enters through various phases of intellectual progression by which the subjects evolves and changes as per the changing dimensions. The knowledge components in the research is updated, modified, changed, accepted or rejected due the contribution of various researches on that subject or area. Every researcher must conduct a thorough review of literature so that the research efforts can be directed towards meaningful contribution to the field of study.

Review of literature requires higher order of abilities where the researcher analyses the existing literature, synthesize the outputs of various researches to develop an understanding and also evaluates the available researches to find out an appropriate plan of action for one's own research. Review of literature is helpful in various ways to the researcher.

- The most important contribution of a review of literature is identification of the research gap on a field of study. It would not only give correct direction to the researcher but the knowledge created through the research will help in filling the existing research gap which is very much needed for the advancement of a discipline.

- The existing knowledge also need to be tested in the light of new paradigms, situations hence review of literature provides an opportunity to provide a fresh interpretation of the previous research work.
- The researcher can frame appropriate research objectives, hypotheses and can select relevant methods and sample on the basis of previous researches.
- A meta-analytic review of literature is especially useful in developing an understanding about the areas or topics where conflicting or contradictory results have been obtained.

2.2 Sources of Review of Literature

The sources of review of literature are the original articles published in both print and electronic forms. The availability of electronic databases have eased and supported the review work and has given access of worldwide researches to the aspiring researchers. Some review research papers which are based on the reviews of the reviews is also very helpful in giving a researcher a better insight on the chosen topic and is also time saving. The sources can also original written work- poem, diaries, court records, interviews, surveys and original research/fieldwork and research published in scholarly/academic journals, dictionaries, encyclopaedia, textbooks and books and articles that interpret, review or synthesize original research/fieldwork.

Indexes- provides citations that fully identify a work with information such as name of the author, titles of a book, articles or journals, publisher and publication date, volume and issue number and page number.

Abstracts- summarize the primary or secondary sources,

Databases- are original indexes that usually include abstracts for each primary or secondary resource and may also include a digital copy of the resource.

2.3 The Present Research

The present research attempts to study the effect of Dance Training and Dance Movement Therapy (DMT) on the personality and psychophysical health of an individual. The present research attempts to emphasize Dance Training/Therapy as it has been proven in different researches that dance training has potential positive effects on physical, mental and emotional well-being. Although the number of researches conducted using DMT as an intervention have been limited in India, that's why the present research will be useful in understanding the role of dance in different psychological variables in Indian context.

2.4 Review of Literature

The reviews of the previous research work have been done in different parts on the basis of dependent variables of the study. The review of literature is focused on the studies conducted on dance training and dance movement therapy and its relationship with the selected dependent variables. The present study has included Personality, Psychophysical health and Anxiety as the dependent variables; hence reviews have been presented separately for these variables. Then the studies of dance movement therapy with other variables have also been presented in the later section.

2.4.1 Research on Personality

University of Haifa, (2020) found that Dance Movement Therapy (DMT) has showed a positive response on bringing physical movements among elderly patients, It also improved quality of life and the familial ties between grandparents and grandchildren. For conducting the study, sixteen dance movement therapists met with their grandmothers for performing three free-form dance sessions. The goal behind these sessions was to determine method by which these sessions would affect each group and how the intergeneration bonds can be strengthen between them. It was seen that initially grandmothers were nervous over their ability to provide a meaningful experience but as they were instructed to see their actions in mirror, encouragement was given regarding their abilities and in between they were provided with rest when they needed, there was more involvement from their side. It was found that elderly populations can improve their physical and mental health and also more connect with their loved ones due to their involvement in dance-movement therapy.

Stephanie (2015) studied that dancers are at high danger of creating cluttered eating mentalities, prominently due to disguised slimness standards. Albeit the large five character characteristics have been demonstrated to be related with eating mentalities in day by day life, in dancers where eating issues and slenderness standards disguise could be remarkable little is thought about these affiliations and the job of the disguise of slimness standards in this relationship The examination included 180 seriously preparing dancers with a normal time of 15.6 years (SD = 2.8). Dancers finished polls estimating the huge five character attributes, disguise of slimness standards and self-guideline of eating mentalities in sport. Bootstrapped intercession examinations showed that neuroticism was contrarily connected with self-guideline of eating perspectives, both straightforwardly and by implication through the intervening job of disguised slenderness standards. This investigation recommended that: (a) neuroticism is a weakness factor for self-guideline of eating perspectives in dancers, as effectively confirmed in everyone, and (b) the disguise of slenderness standards is a pathway through which neuroticism influences self-guideline of eating mentalities. The large five model is along these lines mostly identified with the disguise of slenderness standards and eating mentalities in dancers.

Dinesha & Simpson (2014) studied the relationship between dance movement classes and disruptive behaviour on a sample of 45 at risk students in an urban high school setting. The findings supported the hypothesis that a) dance classes can be utilized as an intervention to reduce stress and b) students who participate in dance programs in public school settings will develop self-control, self-regulation and exhibit less disruptive behaviour.

Alexandros et al. (2012) studied that youth who were involved in dance. The different images were shown on studies regarding effects of dance practices. Most of them referred that dance promotes their personal opportunities, increased levels of socialisation and characteristic behaviour among its participants. The level of socialisation differs according to dance forms and it is also seen that person involves in dance benefitted not only in childhood and adolescence but also were benefitted in adulthood and mature age. The aim of the present review was to provide an overview of major findings of studies concerning the social-physiological outcomes of dance practices, in a general population as well as for adults and adolescents. The typical personality profiles of dancers depended upon the dance form of dancers were relatively high on emotionality strong achievement motivated and exhibits less favourably self-attitudes. Outcomes of dance therapy revealed that better understanding of the true nature of social-psychological outcomes can be provided if specific influential factors are taken into consideration. (i.e.,participants, characteristics, type of guidance, social context and structural qualities of the dance)

Amber & Lynn (2011), studied that individual dance movement therapy is introduced as a modality for healing the wounds of torture. The impact of torture on the body, the self, and relationships, and how this can affect treatment using individual dance movement therapy, was addressed. The author concluded that dance movement therapy, following the experience of torture, can be beneficial in rebuilding an individual's sense of wholeness and self, and in improving interaction skills and relationship capacity.

Shawna (2010) did a theoretical synthesis combining the concepts from Chadian dance/movement therapy and the Responsive Classroom approach to teaching and learning, and suggested a proactive behavioural management style for dance/ movement therapists that incorporated aspects from these two frameworks. For this synthesis, Chadian dance/movement therapy and Responsive Classroom techniques were adapted and implemented. Through combining these two methods, the researcher suggested a unique treatment model as a way to prevent and confront violent and aggressive behaviours of children that were present in a dance/movement therapy session.

Sarah et al. (2006) studied the impact of physical activity on body image dissatisfaction and physical self-perceptions. The research investigated the effects of 6-week aerobic dance on these variables with 50 British schoolgirls aged 13–14 years. A cross-over design was used with two equivalent groups taught normal physical education and aerobic dance in a different order. The Body Attitude Questionnaire (BAQ) and Children and Youth Physical Self-Perception Profile (CY-PSPP) were administered as pre, mid and post-test to each participant in each group before the first intervention, at the changeover and after 12 weeks. The results of this study revealed that participation in 6 weeks of aerobic dance significantly reduced body image dissatisfaction (Attractiveness, Feeling Fat, Salience and Strength and Fitness) and enhanced physical self-perceptions (Body Attractiveness and Physical Self-Worth), although these improvements were not sustained. The implications and future research directions are discussed.

Gronlund & Renck & Weibull (2005) studied a short-term dance movement therapy (DMT) for two young boys with symptoms related to Attention Deficit Hyperactivity Disorder (ADHD). The aim was to investigate the effect and value of DMT as an alternative treatment and to describe the process. The DMT lasted ten sessions and took place once a week during three months. In a case study multiple data sources were used to triangulate the data and describe the DMT process. The DMT has promoted a positive change to a certain extent. DMT provided in paired groups for a minimum of ten weeks will (1) improve the motor function and (2) reduce the behavioural and emotional symptoms of boys aged 5–7 diagnosed with ADHD.

Koshland & Wittaker (2004) examined a 12-week dance movement therapy-based violence prevention program with 54 multicultural elementary school children, and found that it was effective in reducing aggressive behaviours. The program used a dance movement therapy group process that focused on socialization and engagement of children in creative, problem solving experiences. Data showed a decrease in the number of aggressive incidents reported to the principal for the entire school, the decrease in number of incidents for participating classrooms was greater than that for those that did not participate.

Judge et al. (2002) stated that their study reports results of a meta-analysis linking traits from the 5-factor model of personality to overall job satisfaction. Using the model as an organizing framework, 334 correlations from 163 independent samples were classified according to the model. The estimated true score correlations with job satisfaction were -.29 for Neuroticism, .25 for Extraversion, .02 for Openness to Experience, .17 for Agreeableness, and .26 for Conscientiousness. Results further indicated that only the relations of Neuroticism and Extraversion with job satisfaction generalized across studies. As a set, the Big Five traits had a multiple correlation of .41 with job satisfaction, indicating support for the validity of the dispositional source of job satisfaction when traits are organized according to the 5-factor model.

Fern & Meg (1991) studied that dance movement therapy can make to the treatment of battered women. By motivating female victims of domestic violence to act, dance movement therapy addresses patterns of helplessness, ambivalence, and inactivity. Dance movement interventions help women internalize a positive self-concept as well as gain physical and emotional control. In keeping with the short-term, crisis-oriented nature of standard treatment of battered women, a psychosocial plan of intervention which addresses their isolation and immobilization is recommended.

Crain et al. (1983) studied that Educable Mentally Retarded (EMR) adolescents may exhibit problems in social and physical development in comparison with their normal peers. The purpose of this investigation was to study the effects of a 10-week dance program on EMR adolescents. A multiple measurement approach was employed to assess potential effects. Results suggested that nature of participation, consistency of participation, and the design of the curriculum are factors that affect the improvement of social and physical behaviours such as cooperation, dance skills, increased movement repertoire, rhythms, leadership and successful peer teaching.

2.4.2 Research on Anxiety

Vicky et al. (2019) studied that three hundred and fifty-one people with depression (mild to severe) participated, 192 of whom attended DMT groups while receiving treatment as usual (TAU) and 159 received TAU only. Qualitative findings suggest there was a decrease in depression scores in favour of DMT groups in all studies. Subgroup analysis performed on depression scores before and 3 months after the completion of DMT groups suggested changes in favour of the DMT groups. When sensitivity analysis was performed, RCTs at high risk of bias were excluded, leaving only studies with adult clients up to the age of 65. In these studies, the highest effect size was found favouring DMT plus TAU for adults with depression, when compared to TAU only.

Sabine et al.(2019) analysed the intervention of DMT and found that DMT was a significant moderator of results by means of sensitivity analysis. Results thus observed showed that DMT proved to be beneficial in reduction of depression, anxiety and increases quality of life and interpersonal and cognitive skills and the dance interventions shows increase in (psycho) motor skills. Larger effects sizes outcomes from the observational measures might be the reasons behind indicating bias whereas most of the effects remained stable or slightly increased in the follow up data obtained post 22 weeks of the intervention.

Mastura et al. (2015) studied the effect of a 12-week low intensity dance exercise intervention in the treatment of hostility subscale, anxiety subscale and depression subscale among overweight women working in Malaysia in an attempt of Sports for all. It was concluded that low intensity dance therapy exercise intervention of "Aero mass" had contributed greatly to the positive findings concerning physical health and psychological well-being among overweight women in Malaysia.

Sabine et al. (2014), in their studies evaluated the effectiveness of dance movement therapy (DMT) and the therapeutic use of dance for the treatment of health-related psychological problems. Results suggested that DMT and dance are effective for increasing quality of life and decreasing clinical symptoms such as depression and anxiety. Positive effects were also found on the increase of subjective well-being, positive mood, affect, and body image.

Pinniger et al. (2013) observed that DMT and dance are useful in increasing quality of life and also there is decrease in clinical symptoms such as depression and anxiety also there is increase in positive effects is seen an increase of subjective wellbeing, positive mood and body image. The 8 week program was conducted in which 64 participants were assessed before and after 1 month follow up programme was conducted. In this programme the dependent variables like depression, anxiety, stress, fatigue and insomnia and their symptoms were measured. Positive psychology measures were also measured for self-efficacy, satisfaction with life and mindfulness. The scores thus observed were recorded on the control group basis which is discussed here. Group of participants having depression, stress and was not satisfied with life showed benefits by meditation. In the same way participants of exercise group showed decreased depression but the self-efficacy was persistent at post test and the stress was significant at follow up. At post follow-up participants of Tango group had also shown decrease in depression and insomnia and increase in life satisfaction and mindfulness.

Andrea & Karkou & Meekums (2012) studied that depression affects 121 million people worldwide (WHO, 2010). The socio-economic repercussions of depression are putting an enormous strain on UK and US governmental health budgets. Regarding treatment interventions, Dance Movement Therapy and other arts therapies are widely practiced around the world as a treatment of choice for depression. Research evidence suggested that exercise has positive effects on mood. Similarly, it has been argued that dance has a positive social-cultural influence on a person's wellbeing.

Marjolein & Van der (2011), studied that mood can influence our everyday behaviour and people often seek to reinforce, or to alter their mood, for example by turning on music. Music listening while driving is a popular activity. However, little is known about the impact of music listening while driving on physiological state and driving performance. In the present experiment, it was investigated whether individually selected music can induce mood and maintain moods during a simulated drive. In addition, effects of positive, negative, and no music on driving behaviour and physiological measures were assessed for normal and high cognitive demanding rides. Subjective mood ratings indicated that music successfully maintained mood while driving. Narrow lane width drives increased task demand as shown in effort ratings and increased swerving. Furthermore, respiration rate was lower during music listening compared to rides without music, while no effects of music were found on heart rate. Overall, the current study demonstrates that music listening in car influences the experienced mood while driving, which in turn can impact driving behaviour.

Pericleous & Isabella (2011), in his study he focused on the effects of dance movement therapy on people with depression. However, the results have pointed in a positive direction. He believed that if movement therapists as well as psychotherapists pay close attention to this condition, there will be a significant increase in research on using dance to reduce severe depression and melancholia.

Jaclyn (2010) studied the effects of dance therapy and relaxation therapy on anxiety level in college students, 24 undergraduate students from Catholic Liberal Arts College in New England were selected as participants and categorised into two groups. The first group was provided with dance therapy treatment in which students followed an instructor via videotape so to reduce their anxiousness level and the other group was provided with relaxation therapy treatment in which students listened to audio tape which is composed of music that tense and relax muscle group accompanied with deep breathing. The outcome of the study has showed that dance therapy experienced greater decrease in anxiety levels due to processes of self-expression and nonverbal communication which helps students to release their feeling of anxiousness. All students were administered with the Speilberger State-Trait Anxiety Inventory.

Sabine et al. (2007) studied the specific effects of a dance intervention on the decrease of depression and the increase of vitality and positive affect in 31 psychiatric patients with main or additional diagnosis of depression. Patients participated in one of three conditions: a dance group performing a traditional upbeat circle dance, a group that listened just to the music of the dance (music only), and a group that moved on a home trainer bike (ergometer) up to the same level of arousal as the dance group (movement only). While all three conditions alleviated or stabilized the condition of the patients, results suggest that patients in the dance group profited most from the intervention. They showed significantly less depression than participants in the music group ($p < .001$) and in the ergometer group ($p < .05$), and more vitality (p

< .05) than participants in the music group on post-test self-report scales immediately after the intervention. Stimulating circle dances can thus have a positive effect on patients with depression and may be recommended for use in dance/movement therapy and other complementary therapies.

Koch & Morlinghaus & Fuchs (2007) conducted an study on 31 patients with main or additional depression and have shown decrease of depression and increase in vitality and positive effects due to the dance intervention. Patients who participated in any of these three groups out of these groups one was performing traditional dance upbeat in circle manner, second group only listened music (not danced) and third who moved to home on home trainer bike (ergo meter) were aroused to same level as that of dance group (movement only). Results of study indicates that the patients in the group of dance movement were benefitted the most by the intervention as they showed significant reduction in depression in comparison to the patients of music group (p>.001) and to that of patient of ergo meter (p >.05) and more vitality (p >.05) than participants in music group on post-test, self-report immediately after the intervention. These led to the outcome that simulating circle dance can be recommended for use in dance/movement therapy and other complimentary therapies as it shows positive effects on the patients of depression.

Jeong et al. (2005) provided a 12-week Dance Movement Therapy (DMT) program and then assessed the profiles of psychological health and changes in neurohormones of adolescents with mild depression The outcomes has showed that DMT can help in stabilising sympathetic nervous system and it was also seen that DMT can be effective in beneficially modulating concentration of serotonin and dopamine and can improve physiological distress in adolescents with mild depression.

Andre L.& John R. (1990) studied that the effects of modern dance on anxiety. While using the Spielberg State-Trait Anxiety Inventory, state anxiety was assessed before and after 3-month education programme. A class in modern dance was followed by the target group. Three categories of control group are constituted i.e. (1) physical group to control for the effects of exercise. (2). music group to control for aesthetic sensitivity training and (3) a mathematical group. Many factors like age, sex, attitude towards dance and previous experience in dance, sport and relaxation were measured and it is seen that dance therapy reduces anxiety while control activities were unable to do so. On examining concomitant variables, it was concluded that the result could not be accounted for by any obvious artefacts.

2.4.3 Research on Psychophysical Health

Young et al. (2016) studied that dancing is characterised by physical movement in accordance with rhythm perception. Twelve sport dancers and 12 age- and sex-matched young adults who had no dance experience (control group) were recruited. Body intelligence and brain activity were assessed in both groups using the Body Intelligence Scale (BIS) and resting state functional magnetic resonance imaging. BIS scores of dancers were higher than those of control subjects. The dancer group showed increased functional connectivity from the precentral gyrus to the right cingulate gyrus, right occipital fusiform gyrus, right inferior frontal gyrus, right medial frontal gyrus, left inferior frontal gyrus, right parietal postcentral gyrus, and right frontal lobe compared with control subjects. Sport dancers had increased body intelligence sensitivity compared with matched controls. In addition, the characteristics of dance, including physical movement in accordance with rhythm perception, might be associated with increased brain activity in the somato-sensory and rhythm perception networks.

Orsolya et al. (2015) studied that dancing is a popular form of physical exercise and studies have shown that dancing can decrease anxiety, increase self-esteem, and improve psychological wellbeing. The aim of the current study was to explore the motivational basis of recreational social dancing and develop a new psychometric instrument to assess dancing motivation. The sample comprised 447 salsa and/or ballroom dancers (68% female; mean age 32.8 years) who completed an online survey. Eight motivational factors were identified via exploratory factor analysis and comprise a new Dance Motivation Inventory: Fitness, Mood Enhancement, Intimacy, Socialising, Trance, Mastery, Self-confidence and Escapism. Mood Enhancement was the strongest motivational factor for both males and females, although motives differed according to gender. Dancing intensity was predicted by three motivational factors: Mood Enhancement, Socialising, and Escapism. The eight dimensions identified cover possible motives for social recreational dancing, and the DMI proved to be a suitable measurement tool to assess these motives. The explored motives such as Mood Enhancement, Socialising and Escapism appear to be similar to those identified in other forms of behaviour such as drinking alcohol, exercise, gambling, and gaming.

Falisha et al. (2015) studied that dance is a universal form of human expression that offers a rich source for scientific study. Dance provides a unique opportunity to investigate brain plasticity and its interaction with behaviour. Several studies have investigated the behavioural correlates of dance, but less is known about the brain basis of dance. Studies on dance observation suggested that long- and short-term dance training affect brain activity in the action observation and simulation networks. Despite methodological challenges, the feasibility of conducting neuro-imaging while dancing has been demonstrated, and several brain regions have been implicated in dance execution. It was suggested that long-term dance training changes both gray and white matter structure. This article provided a critical summary of work investigating the neural correlates of dance.

Laura et al. (2015) investigated how episodic memory performance can be improved by manipulating the factors that are crucial for successful encoding. There is an ongoing debate about whether a complex stimulus such as music can improve memory, and in particular memory for words, rather than interfere with correct encoding of information. This study aimed to investigate whether verbal episodic memory can be improved by background context of instrumental music. Twenty young adults were asked to memorize different lists of words presented against a background of music, environmental sounds or silence. Their episodic memory performance was then tested in terms of item and source memory scores. Results revealed better memory performance under the music condition than with environmental sounds or silence in the retrieval of the context (i.e. source) of the encoded material. These findings, contrasting with studies showing an interfering effect of music, are discussed in terms of both methodological and theoretical perspectives with the aim of furthering the debate about music and memory. In sum, our results indicate that music can specifically act as a facilitating encoding context for verbal episodic memory, opening important perspectives for music as a rehabilitation tool for episodic memory deficits.

Duim do Nascimento & Silva (2015) studied the functional rehabilitation after a fall involving motor and proprioceptive work as well as being closely connected with psycho-emotional aspects. Dance movement therapy is kind of creative exercise which utilises body in developing this art. After considering studies on dance movement therapy they perform the quasi-experimental study in ten elderly patients for rehabilitation and then they were evaluated on the basis of their quality of life (WHOQOL-Bref), balance (Tinetti Balance Scale- BBS and Berg scale) and mobility (Timed "Up and Go" test-TUG), before and after treatment. Total 16 sessions of therapies was conducted with the goal of creating body self-awareness, spatial perception, co-ordination in relation to song and movement and creativity. Improvement in quality of life has been shown by student's t-test (physical p=0.028, psychological p=0.049, Social p=0.027 and environmental p=0.032). In the same way improvement is seen in balance and mobility with the help of Wilcoxon test (BBS p=0.016; Berg Scale p=0.017, TUG p=0.005). The outcome of the study has supported the theory that dance has positive effect on motor aspects which results in improving mobility and balance and on practicing regularly dance movement therapy in group it can improve quality of life. This study postulates that DMT is beneficial and also low-cost therapy for elderly women who has a history of fall.

Arpita C. (2013) studied that Dance increases total body movement, which helps to improve circulatory, respiratory, skeletal and muscular systems. It has a positive effect on physical health as well as mental and emotional wellbeing. In western world, dance has been used as a form of therapy in many hospitals and medical settings, whether alternate or complementary. The effects of different folk and tribal dance forms of West Bengal on physical, mental and social health are discussed in her study.

Harvard Medical School Department of Neurobiology (2012) studied that the Latin-style dance program known as Zumba improves mood and certain cognitive skills, such as visual recognition and decision-making. Other studies show that dance helps reduce stress, increases levels of the feel-good hormone serotonin, and helps develop new neural connections, especially in regions involved in executive function, long-term memory, and spatial recognition.

Raquel & de (2010) In patients with Multiple Sclerosis (MS) balance and motor coordination within a physiotherapy program when dance was used as therapeutic resource also the patients aided with dance intervention shows the positive effect in neurological function scales (EDSS, NRS, MDS) as they achieved greater postural and balance control. The patient also reported an amelioration of her emotional state. This patient started to perform his previously daily life activities as there was improved physical functioning.

Asmita (2010), Cognitive development is positively affected by the factors of dance therapy which is proven through the result that dance movement therapy create good environment for cognitive development. It is seen that it can be beneficial to the most of the children and can also be implied to maximum number of teachers.

Eva (2004) examined comparative changes in hormonal, emotional, physical and visual status changes in female fibromyalgia (FMS) patients after treatment with Creative Art therapy; dance/movement therapy in comparison with controls. Patients with FMS disorder suffers for chronic pain and the reason behind are musculoskeletal aches, stiffness and pain where perturbations in the stress-axis and high scores on somatic anxiety and muscular tensions also have been found. In this study 36 female FMS patients are included and then divided in two groups which are treatment group and control group. Concentration of hormones in plasma like prolactin, dehydroepiandrostone sulphate (DHEA-S), cortisol and neuropeptide Y (NPY) and of cortisol in saliva were taken and then analysed. Different verbal self-rating scales concerning well-being pain, personality and life events among other things have been used. Patients with FMS syndrome who are affected by video-viewing were assessed and then they were evaluated together with interviews regarding self-perception phenomenon of video viewing (a phenomenal hermeneutic method). It is seen that patients after going through dance/ movement therapy has shown improvement in both psychological and physical functions which is proven by visual analysis. The video interpretation technique (VIT) and self-figure drawing captured treatment that were not evident from verbal scales or reflected in hormonal levels. Biological markers may take longer treatment period to activate the HPA axis and its inter-related hormones and peptides.

McCord, Nichols & Patterson (1989) studied the effects of a 12-week program of low impact aerobic dance conditioning on VO2max, submaximal heart rates and body composition of college-aged women. Sixteen women exercised three times per week for approximately 45 minutes per session at 75-85% of their heart rate reserve. VO2max was measured by indirect calorimetry using a treadmill protocol. Submaximal heart rates were measured by electrocardiography, and body fat was assessed by hydrostatic weight. All testing was conducted within one week pre- and post-training. Training sessions consisted of a 5-10 minute warm up, 30-35 minute low impact aerobic dance segment and a 5 minute cool down. Posttest results revealed a small (7%), but significant increase in VO2max (pre: 38.3 ml/kg/min; post: 41.3 ml/kg/min, X +/- SD, p less than 0.05). Submaximal heart rates at minutes 2-3, 3-4 and 4-5 of the graded exercise test decreased significantly. Body fat decreased from 25 +/- 6.8% to 21 +/- 6.3% (p less than 0.01) with no post training change in body weight. It was concluded that low impact aerobic dance is as effective as other endurance training regimens in improving cardiovascular fitness and decreasing body fat.

2.4.4 Research on dance with other variables

Jordan & Donahue (2020) studied subjective strategies to investigate the encounters of National Grid linemen for the reasons for making a dance development treatment warm-up. Data was accumulated through singular gatherings, where inquiries concerning member's physical, mental and enthusiastic wellbeing were examined comparable to their particular occupation. From the data accumulated, six topics were recognized. To address the perceived issues, eight proposed warm-ups were made. The warm ups, explicitly made from member's firsthand records, are established in both Laban Movement Analysis standards and Bartineff Fundamentals. Meetings are planned to be controlled by an authorized dance development specialist toward the start of every workday and would keep going for roughly 15 minutes. Future ramifications incorporate further exploration, which would investigate the viability and saw advantages of made meetings with line laborers to additionally investigate the advantages of dance movement treatment with the individuals who contain this dedicated population.

Elizabeth (2016) explored methods for bringing dance history directly into the studio. She showed how the movement components that have proven successful in introductory courses can be extended to in-depth studies of dance history with dancers who have formal training. Through the example of a research project on the early work of George Balanchine, it shows how kinaesthetic learners can be introduced to the scholarly side of this art form in a way that shows them its relevance and gives them tools that they can use in their own careers as dancers and choreographers. Finally, she demonstrated how this method allows students the opportunity to explore history through movement in conjunction with archival material, photographs, books, papers and videos.

Hannah et al. (2015) studied that in both partnered Latin dance and non-partnered Latin-themed aerobic dance has increased in recent years, likely a result of the gaining popularity of these types of instructor-led group classes among the mainstream dance and fitness audiences; however, the efficacy of these activities for the purposes of health promotion currently remains unclear. The purpose of this study was to simultaneously assess the physiological responses and psychological experiences during salsa dance and Zumba fitness in a community sample of physically inactive women.

Imogen & Rachel (2015) studied dancers' motivation to work in an independent capacity, and the extent to which dancers' psychological characteristics and skills enabled them to navigate a career in this demanding sector. In-depth semi-structured interviews were conducted with 14 dancers at different stages of their careers. Interviews were transcribed verbatim and content analysed. Analysis revealed that the dancers were intrinsically motivated and highly committed to the profession. Working in the independent sector offered dancers opportunities for growth and fulfilment; they appreciated the autonomy, flexibility and freedom that the independent career afforded, as well as working with new people across roles and disciplines. In order to overcome the various challenges associated with the independent role, optimism, self-belief, social support, and career management skills were crucial. The mental skills reported by the participants had developed gradually in response to the demands that they faced. Therefore, mental skills training could be invaluable for dancers to help them successfully negotiate the independent sector.

Iris (2014) studied that the more than 65 age bunch is continually expanding in size. Asset situated treatment approaches, for example, dance movement treatment (DMT) is getting more significant as they protect the poise of the older, regard their individual requirements and improve social investment. A global web-based study was shipped off 683 DMT partners, of which 113 professionals from Austria, Germany and Switzerland reacted to the accompanying inquiries: To what degree can more established individuals' advantage through DMT? What subjects arise in the meetings? Which restorative intercessions are applied? What are the proposals as to working conditions and the qualities and adapting techniques of specialists? The subjective information investigation uncovers that professionals concur that DMT improves the personal satisfaction of old individuals, encourages support of their connections and extends their assets and cooperation in exercises. The outcomes help us in planning explicit intercession suggestions.

Ho & Rainbow (2014) examined that Breast cancer patients undergoing radiotherapy often suffer from various disease symptoms such as fatigue, pain, and sleep disturbance. These symptoms have been shown to be detrimental to their daily functioning and illness prognosis. The present study aimed to examine the effects of dance movement therapy as an integrated therapeutic intervention on the disease symptoms in breast cancer patients undergoing radiotherapy. The results suggested that dance movement psychotherapy may have therapeutic effects in reducing the pain severity of breast cancer patients receiving radiotherapy.

Iris (2012) conducted a study in which the intervention on quality of life was examined on the basis of the treatment outcome ten weeks dance movement therapy. This whole study was done with design of pre-test, post-test and six month follow up. 162 participants were identified and selected who are suffering from stress were randomly selected and then they were provided with movement therapy treatment group (TG) (n=97) or with wait-listed control group (WG) (65). The significant improvement was seen in psychological domain, social relations, global health, physical health and general life while in long term dance movement therapy shows great improvement in the psychological domain, spirituality and general which leads to draw the conclusion that dance movement therapy is beneficial in short as well as long term in improving quality of life.

Kiepe & Stockigt & Kiel (2012) conducted a study that dance movement therapy has a positive impact for patients with breast cancer, improving quality of life, shoulder range of motion and body image. In patients with depression psychological distress was reduced by dance therapy. Ballroom dance improved balance and coordination in patients with Parkinson's disease and disease-specific quality of life in patients with heart failure. Dance movement therapy and ballroom dance seem beneficial for patients with breast cancer, depression, Parkinson's disease, diabetes and heart failure.

Michelle (2010) considered what movement therapist does and how their administrations connect with traditional psychotherapy. The motivation behind this venture was to give data about dance movement treatment as an approach to advance the training and move towards overcoming any issues between this elective treatment and standard psychotherapies. This exploratory and spellbinding examination was brought out through semi-organized meetings. The sample (N=9) was made of up dance movement specialist who were ensured by the American Dance Therapy Association. Questions were intended to accumulate data about members segment, preparing and accreditation cycle, strategies and meaning of dance development treatment, customer qualities and building client base and report. A substance examination of discoveries showed that dance movement specialist does encounter challenges in building up an affinity inside the psychological well-being field. It was likewise found that the vast majority have a helpless comprehension of what dance movement treatment is and how it functions as psychotherapeutic treatment. Social and profound ramifications are inspected too, as they identify with the elective act of dance development treatment.

Emily (2010), This qualitative research explored creative movement processes such as dance movement therapy (DMT), authentic movement (AM), and creative dance (CD) as possible tools for transforming sexual trauma for women. Eleven movement professionals were interviewed in a semi-structured research format. Her direct experience and knowledge of sexual abuse, sexual trauma, and creative movement processes were interwoven with the research question: Do creative dance movement therapy processes contribute to the dynamic of healing for women transforming sexual trauma? These findings were inconclusive for the greater population of survivors of sexual abuse and sexual trauma. However, there were indications that DMT, AM, and CD may be potential tools for recovery. This research contributed to a dialogue about sexual abuse and recovery from sexual trauma.

Than et al. (2010)A nonpharmacological method can be an alternative or complement to analgesics. The aim of this study was to evaluate if music medicine influences pain and anxiety in children undergoing lumbar punctures. A randomized clinical trial was used in 40 children (aged 7-12 years) with leukaemia, followed by interviews in 20 of these participants. The participants were randomly assigned to a music group (n = 20) or control group (n = 20). The primary outcome was pain scores and the secondary was heart rate, blood pressure, respiratory rate, and oxygen saturation measured before, during, and after the procedure. Anxiety scores were measured before and after the procedure. Interviews with open-ended questions were conducted in conjunction with the completed procedures. The results showed lower pain scores and heart and respiratory rates in the music group during and after the lumbar puncture. The anxiety scores were lower in the music group both before and after the procedure. The findings from the interviews confirmed the quantity results through descriptions of a positive experience by the children, including less pain and fear.

Tomas et al. (2010) studied that the relationship between individual differences and specific uses of music, referring to why and how people use music in everyday life. Questionnaire data from 341 respondents showed that open and intellectually engaged individuals, and those with higher IQ scores, tended to use music in a rational/cognitive way, while neurotic, introverted and non-conscientious individuals were all more likely to use music for emotional regulation (e.g. change or enhance moods). Results suggest that individual differences in personality and cognitive ability may partly determine the way in which we experience music. Limitations and suggestions for future studies are discussed

Wiley (2008) reported that the British Government had taken initiatives to include dance in promoting social and educational inclusion through arts on the basis of the results of the researches which had shown the relationship between the social classes of peoples. On analysing data it was seen that attitudes to aspects of dance varies with social class and that there was interaction between gender and social class in just one instance. The major outcome of the study was that the maximum number of children in schools should be benefited by the dance arts and also young people can have reach to aesthetic experiences that have potential to improve quality of life. It was concluded that the current limited provision within the national curriculum may be contributing to the social and educational exclusions of some pupils.

Watson & Dr Garrett (2006) of the University of Hertfordshire compared members of the Royal Ballet with a squad of British national and international swimmers. In their research, they found that the dancers scored higher than the swimmers in seven out of ten areas of fitness.

Marika & Samantha (2000) investigated the relationship between amount of exercise and psychological well-being in a broadly based sample. A questionnaire assessing amount of exercise, reasons for exercise, body satisfaction, and self-esteem was completed by 252 participants between the ages of 16 and 60 years. Participants were divided into four groups on the basis of gender and age, resulting in 70 young women, 48 young men, 73 mature women, and 61 mature men. Significant negative relationships between amount of exercise and body satisfaction and self-esteem were found for young women, and positive relationships for the remainder of the sample. Women exercised more for reasons of weight control, tone, and mood enhancement than men. For the whole sample, the first two of these reasons were associated with lower body satisfaction, while exercising for health and fitness reasons was associated with increased self-esteem. It was concluded that reasons for exercising did not provide an adequate explanation for the obtained difference in correlations across gender and age.

2.4.5 Synthesizing Reviews

The above review of literature has shown that the effect of dance and dance movement therapy has been studied on the variety of sample. The chosen sample in these researches has included the elderly population, children undergoing lumbar punctures, women who have experienced sexual trauma, dance movement specialist, patients with breast cancer, adolescents and adults who were suffering from stress, female with fibromyalgia, the patients who have Multiple Sclerosis (MS), the individuals who were undergoing functional rehabilitation after a fall, salsa and/or ballroom dancers, patients with anxiety and depression, Educable Mentally Retarded (EMR) persons and the female victims of domestic violence etc.

Dance movement therapy and dance training has been found to be effective for healing the wounds of torture, in reducing aggressive behaviours among elementary school children, in controlling the symptoms of depression and other mood disorders, in improving the physical fitness, in controlling the behavioural and emotional symptoms shown by the patients diagnosed with ADHD. It has also been found effective in developing self-control, self-regulation and in exhibiting less disruptive behaviour among at risk students. Some researchers have focused on the specific dance forms such as Zumba, Salsa and Ballroom dance etc.

2.5 Research Gap

On the basis of the above review of literature, some major **research gaps** have been identified in the proposed field of investigation.

There are fewer researches which has compared the psychological profiles of dancers and non-dancers. There are researches conducted on various samples as discussed above, the researchers comparing the adolescents on the basis of their involvement in dance training is missing.

It is also missing whether the usual dance training, which focuses on the steps, skills, acts, performance differs, differs from the therapeutic use of dance. The comparison of dance trainees and non-dance trainees and using the dance movement therapy as an intervention in the same research are also missing.

Various studies have been conducted on psychological and physical factors of dance movement therapy like effect of DMT on Depression, Cancer, Dementia, Autism but only few empirical studies are available which have studied the personality traits of dancers and how the personality traits of dancers differ from non-dancers. The present research has chosen to study the big five personality traits among dancer and then compare these personality traits with non-dancers.

Both Physical and Mental health has been an important facet of an individual's quality of life; hence present research has included psychophysical health as a variables in the study. Empirical studies on psychological and physical health related to Dance Movement Therapy in India are very few

The researches focusing the effect of DMT on anxiety in Indian contests are available but are limited in number to develop a comprehensive picture. Such researches are scantily found in the geographical area chosen for the study.

CHAPTER - 3

METHOD AND PROCEDURE

Research methodology consists of the plan, structure and the strategy a researcher adopts for conducting a research. It is important for a research to come up with the findings that are applicable on the larger groups, the intended population. Research techniques and methods are important in accuracy of the outcomes we get from the research. The techniques and system are viewed as the foundation of any exploration. This chapter gives a detailed view of the methods, tools and techniques used by the researcher

The researcher outlines research goals keeping in view the information and knowledge that one has accomplished during the time spent studying the current writings on the subject selected for the research. Survey of Literature is additionally valuable for selecting an appropriate topic for the exploration. Based on these bits of knowledge, the researcher chooses strategies from among the accessible alternatives.The researcher readies the research framework and plan, how the sample would be chosen, which techniques would be utilized for choosing test, which factors would be chosen for study, which information assortments strategies and instruments would be generally fitting for the chosen factors, what might be the scoring systems, how the information would be investigated with proper insights according to the idea of the information and so on.

Thus, it tends to be said as characterized by different analysts that methodology relates to the arrangement, structure and technique planned in order to get answer to the research questions. It also identified the control factors and makes appropriate plan to control these factors so that the precise relationships for the targeted variables can be understood and the effect of extraneous variables can be controlled. The methodology incorporates a total layout of what the researcher did from composing the speculations and their operational ramifications to the last investigation of the information.

3.1 OBJECTIVES

The title of the present research is 'Personality & Psychophysical Health in relation to Dance Training: A Therapeutic Intervention of Dance Movement Therapy'. After conducting an extensive review of literature, the following research objectives and hypotheses were framed:

1. To study the effect of Dance Training on personality (Openness, Conscientiousness, Extraversion, Agreeableness and Neuroticism), level of anxiety & psychophysical health
2. To study the effect of gender on an individual's personality, level of anxiety & psychophysical health
3. To study the interaction effect of gender (male & female) and dance training (dance trainee & non dance trainee) on personality, level of anxiety & psychophysical health
4. To prepare an intervention model based on Dance Movement Therapy
5. Therapeutic intervention of Dance Movement Therapy to study its effect on personality, level of anxiety & psychophysical health

3.2 HYPOTHESES

1. There is no difference between the personality of Dance Trainee and Non-Dance Trainee.
2. There is no difference between the psychophysical health of Dance Trainee and Non-Dance Trainee.
3. There is no difference between the level of anxiety of Dance Trainee and Non-Dance Trainee.
4. There is no difference between the personality of Males and Females.
5. There is no difference between the psychophysical health of Males and Females.
6. There is no difference between the level of anxiety of Males and Females.
7. There is no effect of therapeutic use of dance movement therapy on personality, psychophysical health and anxiety.

3.3 VARIABLES

Dance Training and Gender have been selected as the independent variables for the present research. Dance Training has two categories Dance Trainee and Non-Dance Trainee. Gender also has two categories Male and Female.

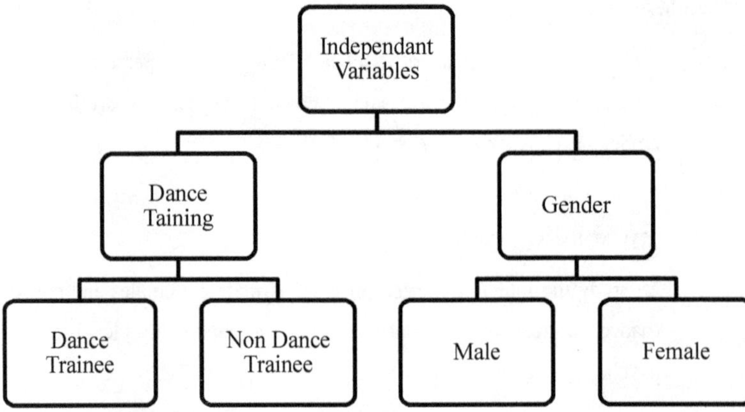

The following three variables were selected as dependents variables for the present research.

a. Personality – Big five traits

   (Openness, Conscientiousness, Extraversion, Agreeableness and Neuroticism)

b. Psychophysical Health (Mental and Physical health)

c. Anxiety

3.4 RESEARCH DESIGN

The present research was conducted in two phases. In the first phase, the research collected data from the sample of 120 adolescents selected as per the factorial design shown below. In the second phase, the research conducted dance-movement therapy on 20 adolescents divided in two groups; one control and one experimental group.

<u>Phase I</u>

A total sample of 120 adolescents was selected as per the 2x2 factorial design.

Table 3.1 : 2x2 factorial design (Phase-I)

	Dance Trainee (B_1)	Non-Dance Trainee (B_2)	Total
Male (A_1)	A_1B_1 (N=30)	A_1B_2 (N=30)	60
Female (A_2)	A_2B_1 (N=30)	A_2B_2 (N=30)	60
Total	60	60	120

There were four groups as per the factorial design.

Group 1: Male adolescents who are receiving dance training (N=30)

Group 2: Male adolescents who are NOT receiving dance training (N=30)

Group 3: Female adolescents who are receiving dance training (N=30)

Group 4: Female adolescents who are NOT receiving dance training (N=30)

Phase II

Dance Movement Therapy Intervention

An intervention model based on the dance-movement therapy principles and techniques was prepared by the researcher. The specific techniques, number of sessions, its sequence and duration were decided to finalise an intervention model. This intervention model was used by the researcher to provide dance-movement therapy to selected adolescents in Phase-II of the research.

A Before-After Two group Control-Experimental Design was used for the Phase-II therapeutic sessions. A sample of 20 adolescents was selected randomly from 60 adolescents from Phase-I. These adolescents had never received any dance training and were a part of non-dance trainee group.. Their pre-test data on Personality, Mental Health and level of Anxiety was already available.

Table 3.2: Before-After Two Groups Design (Phase II)

Group	Pre-test	Intervention	Post-test
Control Group (N=10)	• Personality • Psychophysical health • Anxiety	No Intervention	• Personality • Psychophysical health • Anxiety
Experimental Group (N=10)	• Anxiety Personality • Psychophysical health • Anxiety	Intervention (Dance Movement Therapy)	• Personality • Psychophysical health • Anxiety

The selected 20 adolescents were randomly assigned to different groups to form two groups. To assign the treatments randomly, which group would serve as the control group and which group would serve as experimental group was also decided randomly. After formation of control and experimental groups, the experimental group was provided dance-movement therapy (DMT) as per the sessions and duration specified in the intervention model prepared by the researcher. The control group was not provided dance-movement therapy.

Once the DMT intervention was complete, post-testing for anxiety, psychophysical health and personality was done to get the comparative score to analyse the effect of DMT on the three dependent variables.

3.5 SAMPLE

Locale

The locale of the present study was confined to Udaipur district of Rajasthan. The sample was selected from the different Dance Institutes of Udaipur. The sample of non-dancers is also taken from Udaipur district.

Sample

The sample comprised of 120 adolescents out of which 60 adolescents were receiving dance training and the remaining 60 adolescents have not received any dance training. The adolescents who have received dance training have been referred to as 'Dance trainees' (DT) in the present research. The adolescents who have not received any type of dance training have been referred as 'non-dance trainees' (NDT) in the present research. In each of the DT and NDT group, equal numbers of male and female adolescents were selected in the sample. That means, in each group, there were 30 male and 30 female adolescents selected as per the factorial design of the research discussed earlier. The sample was selected from different dance Institutes of Udaipur district in Rajasthan in Phase-I. In Phase-II, 20 adolescents selected randomly from non-dance trainee group of Phase-I were selected.

A list was created by including male and female learners in the age range between 18-30 years from different dance institutes of Udaipur. 30 boys and 30 girls were selected randomly from that list to be a part of 'dance trainee' group.

Inclusion criteria: In this study, adolescents of age group 18-30 years, who have undergone at least 3 months of dance training, were selected as Dance Trainees.

Exclusion criteria: Samples below the age group 18 and above the age 30 were not be included.

SAMPLING PLAN

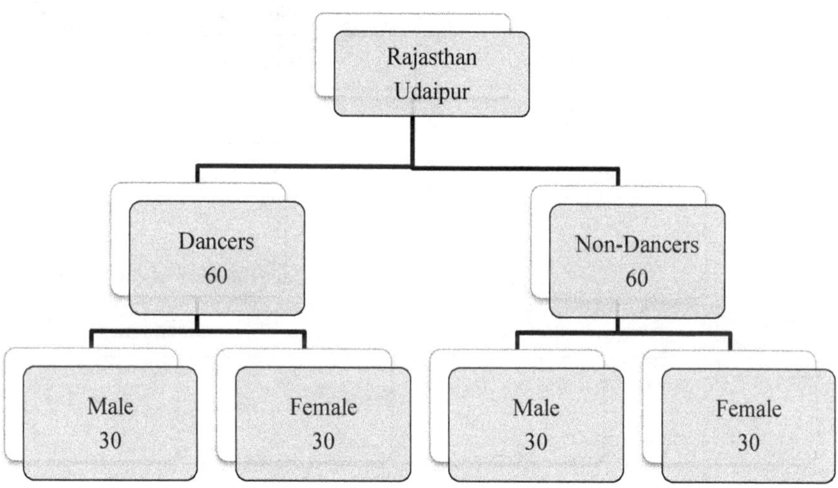

3.6 DEMOGRAPHIC PROFILE OF THE SAMPLE

The following information related to demographic factors was also collected during data collection. The respondents were asked to fill a Personal Data Sheet along with the tools used for dependent variables of the study.

- Name
- Age
- Gender
- Education
- School/College
- Marital Status
- Dance Trainee or Non-Dance Trainee
- Name of Dance Trainee Institute, if any
- Duration of dance raining

Table 3.3 : Age-wise Classification of Sample

Categories	Frequency	Percent
18-21 years	62	51.7
22-25 years	42	35.0
26-30 years	16	13.3

Table 3.4 : Education-wise Classification of the Sample

Categories	Frequency	Percent
Secondary/ Senior Secondary	14	11.7
Graduation	73	60.8
Post Graduation	33	27.5
Total	120	100.0

3.7 PSYCHOLOGICAL TESTS USED FOR DATA COLLECTION

According to Anastasi and Urbina, psychological tests involve observations made on a "carefully chosen sample of an individual's behavior. They are useful to measure unobserved constructs. The tools are an important elements of any research. The tools used in a research should be standardized so that the results obtained are more reliable. A test shall have the folowing characteristics of a Psychological test- Standardization, Objectivity, Test Norms, Reliability and Validity.

The present research attempts to study the effect of Dance Training and Dance Movement Therapy (DMT) on the personality and psychophysical well-being of an individual. The effect of Dance on Personality, Anxiety and Psychophysical health were studied. The following tools were used for collecting Data-

Table 3.4 : Psychological tests/tools used for Data Collection

Variable	Name of the Test/Scale	Author
Personality	Big Five personality test	Costa & McCrae, 1992
Anxiety	Sinha Anxiety Scale	D. N. Sinha, 1976
Psychophysical health	P.G.I. Health Questionnaire	S K Verma, 1971

3.7.1 Big Five Personality Test-

The NEO Five-Factor Inventory is used for assess personality on five dimensions i.e. are Neuroticism, Extraversion, Openness, Agreeableness, and Conscientiousness. This inventory has a number of versions like240, 180, 96 or 60 items inventory. However, the most applicable to the study carried out, is the 60 items inventory, with least number of responses, within a 5-point scale and the same is described below-

a) **Neuroticism (N)-** It means adjustment or emotional stability with maladjustment or neuroticism. It is the experience of negative feeling such as embarrassment, fear, guilt, sadness etc. High scores in Neuroticism means less able to control their impulses and unable to cope with stress. The individuals who score low on Neuroticism are emotionally stable.

b) **Extraversion (E)-** Extraversion means quantity and intensity of interpersonal interactions, activity level, need for stimulation and capacity for joy. High scores on this dimension tends to be sociable, active, talkative, person oriented, optimistic, fun loving. Low scores show personality of reserved nature, sober, un-exuberant, aloof, task oriented, retiring and quiet.

c) **Openness (O)-** This term includes proactive seeking and appreciation of experience for its own sake; toleration for and exploration of the unfamiliar. High scores on this scale are curious, having broad interests, creative, original, and imaginative. Low scores tend to be conventional, down to earth, with narrow interests, un-artistic and un-analytical.

d) **Agreeableness (A)-** how effectively you get on with different people is calculated by this dimension. High scores on this dimension indicate expected to be a soft hearted, good nurtured, trusting, helpful and forgiving. Low scores show rude, suspicious, uncooperative, irritable and manipulative.

e) **Conscientiousness (C)-** This term evaluates how a person is motivate towards his goal, the degree of his determination. High scores mean hardworking, organized, reliable, punctual, self-discipline etc. Low scores indicate aimless, unreliable, lazy, careless, negligent and hedonistic.

Scoring-

N: If scored below 13 it means low (and below 6 very low) on N and if scored above 21 it means high on N. Otherwise, scored in average range.

E: If scored below 24 (below 18 very low) it means low on E. If scored above 30 (above 36 very high) it means high on E. Otherwise scored in average range.

O: If scored 23 it means low on O (below 18 very low). Above 30 high on O (above 36 very high). Otherwise you scored in average range.

A: If you scored below 29 (below 24 very low) it means low on A. If scored above 35 it means high on A. (and above 40 very high). Otherwise scored in average range.

C: If scored below 30 it means low on C. (below 25 very low). If scored above 37 you are high on C (above 43 very high). Otherwise scored in average range.

a) Reliability- "The reliability of the NEO-FFI had been established by evaluating the Cronbach's-alpha reliability coefficients. The value of the coefficient is 0.90, 0.78, 0.76, 0.86 and 0.90 for the dimensions of neuroticism, extraversion, openness, agreeableness and conscientiousness, respectively. These values are high enough (0.76 and more) to reflect on the reliability of the inventory."

3.7.2 PGI Health Questionnaire-

Directions for Administration and Scoring-

"If the respondent can read Hindi give him/her the test sheet and a pencil. Ask him to put atick against questions he agrees with. Most of the respondents are able to finish this test within 5 minutes. The number of ticks on section A and B indicate the respective scores, which can be then added up to give a total score also.

If the respondent is illiterate, read to him/her each question slowly and record his/her response. If a respondent does not understand the question repeat it or briefly explain it. Avoid long explanations and suggestions on how to reply. Unsophisticated respondents often say things which they think are expected of them and not what they genuinely feel. This test will be useful only if one is able to record what respondent genuinely feels about himself/herself. One's own suggestions should be strictly avoided.

There is no fixed number of questions above which all neurotics should score on this test but in our studies of over 500 persons we found that if a person ticks more than 10 items, chances are high that he has got marked neurotic trends.

A high score need not always indicate neurosis, but (a) it shows a propensity to develop neurotic symptoms under stress, and (b) neurotic scores higher than normal. Some of the 'normals' do develop symptoms later and a few neurotics tend to deny the presence of symptoms which may be considered as socially undesirable responses. Use of a lie scale in addition to it, may prove useful, although the correlations with lie score of the present scale are found low."

3.7.3 Sinha Anxiety Scale-

A test was developed which could tap the different areas or dimensions as well as forms of manifestations of anxiety because manifestation of anxiety is multi-dimensional.

So, questions were drafted to bring out self-ratings on items definitive of anxiety reactions to the subsequent areas:

- Health, appearance and injury.
- Area of ambition.

- Family anxieties
- Anxieties regarding friendship and love
- Social relations and social approval
- Worries regarding the future
- Worries about civilization, war, virtue
- Guilt and shame
- Physical and physiological manifestation
- Purely psychological manifestation

The Self-Analysis form, which is a preliminary form of test, had a total of 140 items of theYes/No type.

Reliability

As determined by the Table, both split-half and test and retest methods had high reliability. It was found that the Standard error of measurement was 6.10 which shows that the true score didn't diverge way too much from the true value.

Table 3.5: Sinha Anxiety Scale Reliability

Method	N	r	Index of reliability	S. E. m.
Split-half	239	.86	.92	6.10
Test-retest	88	.73	.85	

Validity

The count on the Taylor's MAS as amended by the author, was used as the first validation criterion. Taylor's MAS was administered on all the 70 subjects who had taken the test. The correlation that was measured on the unrevised version of the scale was of the similar value as of the test which was .69 which indicated that the two tests were measuring almost the similar

3.8 PROCEDURE OF DATA COLLECTION-

3.8.1 Phase-I

Data were collected through individual face to face interaction. The data collection was done in year 2019. The data was collected at the time of the convenience of the respondents. A comfortable environment was provided to the respondents by establishing proper rapport with them. The purpose of the research was explained during the rapport building process. They were informed about the purpose of the study and their consent for participation in the study was obtained. They were ensured about the confidentiality of the information that they provided. It was also informed that the obtained information will be used only for the research purpose. The personal details like their name and other information will be kept confidential. They were also asked if they had any queries with reference to the research. The respondent's permission was obtained to start the data collection process.

The sets of Personality test, Anxiety Scale and P.G.I. health questionnaire were given to them one by one. They were also instructed to fill their personal information sheet on the front page. The instructions used specifically for various tests and tools used in the research have been given below.

Instructions of the Big-five Personality Test-

"Write only where indicated in this item booklet. Carefully read all of the instructions before beginning. This questionnaire contains 60 statements. Read each statement carefully. For each statement, fill in the circle with the response that best represents your opinion. Make sure that your answer is in the correct box.

Fill in SD if you strongly disagree or the statement is definitely false.

Fill in D if you disagree or the statement is mostly false.

Fill in N if you are neutral on the statement, if you cannot decide, or if the statement is about equally true and false.

Fill in A if you agree or the statement is mostly true.

Fill in SA if you strongly agree or the statement is definitely true.

Note that the responses are numbered in rows.

Fill in only one response for each statement. Respond to all of the statement, making sure that you fill in the correct response. DO NOT ERASE! If you need to change an answer, make an X through the incorrect response and then fill in the correct response.

Before responding to the statement, turn to the inside of this Item Booklet and enter your name, age, sex, ID number (if any) and today's date."

Instructions of Sinha Anxiety Scale-

"There are some sentences related to your social and behavioral problems. These sentences are related to your day to day problems and experience. These sentences are not related to your intelligence test but to the test of some facts. Read carefully every problem. In front of every sentences there are 2 options 'yes' and 'No'. Tick mark the appropriate option according to your situation and behavior. You are totally free to fill the list. Your answer will be kept confidential. It is compulsory to answer all the questions."

Instructions of P.G.I. Health Questionnaire-

"There are some questions related to physical and mental health. Read carefully and tick mark those sentences which are appropriate for you."

3.8.2 Phase-II

Intervention Model

The following Dance Movement Therapy Intervention Model was prepared and used by the researcher in Phase-II. The sessions were provided for four-weeks duration. In each week, various techniques explained below were used by the researcher.

Table 3.6: Dance Movement Therapy Intervention Model

Week	Time	Techniques Used
First week	45 minutes per day	1. Warm-up 2. Dance 3. Stretching
Second week	45 minutes per day	1. Warm-up 2. Jumping with Music 3. Stretching 4. Breathing Exercise 5. Group Technique
Third week	45 minutes per day	1. Warm-up 2. Dance on Melodic music 3. Dance in Circle 4. Movement with props 5. Breathing Exercise 6. Stretching 7. Mirroring
Fourth week	45 minutes per day	1. Warm-up 2. Dance on Fast music 3. Movements in circle 4. Movements with props 5. Breathing exercise 6. Stretching 7. Mirroring

Dance Movement Therapy Techniques

Some techniques used in the intervention model have been explained below.

Warm-up – Warm-up is important to increase the body's core temperature, it also increasing the body's muscle temperature. Increasing muscle temperature is helpful to make the muscles flexible, nimble and malleable. A productive warm up also has the effect of increasing both heart rate and respiratory rate. This increases blood flow, which in turn increases the delivery of oxygen and nutrients to the working muscles. All this helps to prepare the muscles, tendons and joints for more strenuous activity. It includes- Head up and down, shoulder movement (both sides), both hands movement (both sides), waist movement (clock wise and anti-clock wise), legs movement, toes movement, jogging, walking on place etc.

Dance -After warm-up, Bollywood- Freestyle dance was done. Here, participants copied the therapist's dance moves. Therapist was doing dance steps and all were coping her steps. This was very fantastic session. Dance moves includes legs-hands movement, waist movements, it includes whole body movements. Those movements were done on randomly selected Bollywood songs.

Stretching- Stretching is the process of physical health and fitness it includes set down specific parts of the body into a position that will lengthen, or elongate, the muscles and associated soft tissues. Through regular stretching practice a number of changes start to occur within the body and specifically within the muscles themselves. Other tissues that start to adapt to the stretching process include the fascia, tendons, ligaments, skin and scar tissue.

Breathing exercise- In this exercise therapist practiced inhalation and escalation of breath. The therapist's instructions were "Let your Breath flow as deep down into your belly, without forcing it. Try breathing in through your nose and breathing out through mouth. Breathe in gently and regularly. Let it flow out gently."

Jumping with Music- Jumping is such a great exercise to reduce stress. Here, in the session Therapist made them jump in different sides like front jump, back jump, side jump on different tracks of music. The all participants were enjoying this jumping technique.

Group Technique-Group technique is where all members of session move in group. Therapist gave instructions to make a big circle and doing movements in circle as therapist was doing.

They all were moving in circle dancing in circle, doing different movements as therapist was doing. This group technique is useful to promote social well-being. It is beneficial to enhance social ability, cooperation, helping others, coordinate with others and ability to understand other's emotions.

Movement with props- In this technique therapist used different props like colorful ribbons and 'dupatta' in dance. Therapist and participants all were dancing on song with those props. These props lead happiness in participants. All participants were feeling joy and excitement by using those props. This joy and happiness are good for their mental health.

Mirroring- This technique is good to enhance emotional understanding and empathy for others. It this technique therapist imitate the movements of clients, their emotion and their intentions. This technique is commonly practiced in order to enhance empathy of the therapist for the client.

Instructions during DMT Intervention

The movements of this session were followed by some instructions. There were some instructions given by Therapist during session. These instructions were changed according to the sessions. These instructions were given when jumping and breathing exercises were conducted with movements:

"Bend your knees so they are released. Focus on your breath, notice how your body moves with your breath, move slowly, this is your body, you exist, find joy in bounce, bounce, bounce, you can play. When was the last time you jumped? Moves like nobody watching you, you are free totally free, move your spine, feel your spine, feel your heartbeat, its faster, you are alive, breathe, breathe deep breath, release your shoulder, find your inner rhythm, follow me, feel the movements, be brave, it doesn't matter how it all looks, take risks, just follow me. Refresh, follow me, feel your every movement, what are you holding in your hands, bring your negative world, can you compress them, can you crush them, I am crushing my negative vibes, this is my way, now they are dust, they are only thoughts, see how it feels to move this way on all the dust of negative words, I am crushing my negative words with my feet, give love to your body, you have healing power, breathe deep breathe, everything is alright, now we are focusing on our positive world, be focused on your positive thoughts, move with me, just follow me, draw the line of positivity, remember all positive words your positive thoughts, you are happy, you are very happy, you can tolerate everything, you can face everything, be prepare for every situation, just follow me, follow my moves, remember all love you gave your body, you are line, you are love, you are enough, you are a tree that can dance, that can move, move move, refresh, water heals your touch heals, give love to yourself, to your body, move through each parts to see it is okay, how did it change with movement, how did it change with words and exercises, today you gave the time yourself, thanks yourself, love yourself, deep breath and sit on the floor close your eyes feel your breathe, feel your body's energy, calm down feel the peace and relax."

3.9 ETHICAL ISSUES

- Informed Consent and Voluntary Participation: The dance trainee and non-dance trainee were informed about the study. They all knew about objectives of the study.
- Proper Rapport was established before the data collection for both the phases of the research.
- It was ensured that the confidentiality of the given information would be maintained.
- The researcher herself handled the psychological care and support during the data collection.
- The control group in the phase-II was also provided the dance movement therapy after the post-testing was over to offer similarity of treatment/benefits to the adolescents who had not received the DMT intervention earlier.

3.10 ANALYSIS OF DATA

The total scores for every scale for each respondent were obtained for all 120 adolescents after the data was over. For scoring procedures, the test manual of each of the Big Five Personality Test, Sinha Anxiety Scale and PGI Health Questionnaire was followed. After that, the data was entered into Microsoft Excel data sheet. The data which was entered included the demographic profile information as well the total scoress for all 120 people. Mean, S.D. and ANOVA were used for analyzing the data obtained in Phase-I and paired sample t-test was used to compare the control and experimental group in Phase-II.

For analyzing the data, Statistical Package for Social Scientists (SPSS) was used. For comprehending and interpreting the data, following statistical techniques were used.

Mean and Standard Deviation

The mean and standard deviation for personality and its big five traits, anxiety and psycho-physical health were obtained for adolescents dance trainees & non dance trainees. Similarly, the mean and standard deviation for personality, anxiety and psycho-physical health were obtained for male and female adolescents. For the ease of reading and understanding, Mean and S.D. were also presented graphically.

Analysis of Variance (ANOVA)

Analysis of Variance (ANOVA) is a compilation of statistical models and their correlated estimation procedures (like the "variation" among and between groups) used to figure out the differences among group means in a sample. ANOVA is useful in examining the main as well as the interaction of variables. Researchers have selected two independent variables, Gender and Dance Trainee, in the present research. ANOVA has enabled the research in studying the individual effects of each of the independent variables as well as the interaction effect of Gender and Dance Trainee on various dependent variables. A 2 x 2 factorial design has been used in this research to select samples; a two-way factorial ANOVA is appropriate for such types of designs. The p-value was calculated for the three dependent variables and was used for interpreting the level of significance for main as well as interactions effects.

t-test

To compare the mean of two groups, a statistical test called t-test is used. This test is generally used in hypothesis testing to know whether a treatment or process has an effect on the population of interest or whether one group is different from another. t-test is only used to compare the mean of 2 groups. Here, a paired sample t-test was used to as the same groups were pre and post tested on the variables.

CHAPTER 4

RESULT AND DISCUSSION

Result and Discussion section of any research is considered to be the most interesting yet a challenging task for the researcher. During this stage, all the efforts of the researcher; starting from selecting a relevant topic and determining research objectives till the scoring and analysis of the data; come to fruition. The researcher is also keen in finding out what are the main findings of the research.

Results section is focused on the main findings or direct answers to the research questions, mainly consisting of the statistical components. The detailed presentation of results in the form of tables and graphs leads to a better reader friendly presentation. Discussion completes the incomplete by explaining and interpreting the obtained findings, it finds out the meaning of the obtained results, why these results might have occurred, what are the contextual factors responsible, what are its supportive and contradictory findings etc.

A researcher can adopt various approaches while writing this chapter. Simultaneously presenting results and then explaining and discussing these results then and there so that it provides an opportunity to better relate and understand the findings. In this chapter, first results are presented in the form of tables and graphs which are followed by the discussion of the findings. In the discussion, the researcher puts own thought in making the findings more comprehensive. Discussion is looking at the results from more analytical, critical and interpretative perspective so that the final conclusions can be extracted from the research output. Conclusions are further the summary of the discussion which tells us what we learnt from the research. Drawing conclusions is more about winding up and giving a final touch to the obtained knowledge through the process of analysis, interpretation, synthesis, and evaluation. The conclusions of the present research work will be presented in the form of main findings separately in Chapter-6 : Summary.

4.1 OVERVIEW OF THE RESEARCH

This research has been conducted in two phases. In the first phases, 120 persons in the age group 18-30 years (with the mean age approximate 22 years) consisting of 60 dancers and 60 non-dancers were selected and were termed Dance Trainee (DT) and Non-dance Trainee (NDT) group. In each of the two groups, 30 male and 30 female were selected as per the 2 x 2 factorial designs. All the persons were administered with the selected tools to measure their Personality, Psychophysical health and the level of Anxiety.

In the second phase, 20 persons were selected from the NDT group and were randomly assigned to two groups; each group included 10 persons. It was also randomly decided which group would receive the treatment; hence control group and experimental group were also randomly decided. The experimental group was provided the Dance Movement Therapy (DMT) on the basis of Intervention Model prepared by the researcher. The effect of DMT intervention was studied on the Personality, Psychophysical health and the level of Anxiety.

4.2 FINDINGS OF THE STUDY

The findings of the present research were obtained by using various statistical techniques discussed in chapter-3. The findings are presented separately for both the phases of the research; Phase-I and Phase-II.

Phase-I

In this phase, the obtained results on the following variables from 120 persons have been discussed variable-wise.

1. Personality
2. Anxiety
3. Psychophysical health

4.2.1 Personality:

4.2.1.1 Frequency Distribution: NEO-Five Factors

Table 4.1: Different levels of Personality factors (NEO-FFI)

Level of Personality	Neuroticism	Extraversion	Openness	Agreeableness	Conscientiousness
Very high	Above 29	Above 36	Above 36	Above 40	Above 43
High	22-29	31-36	31-36	36-40	38-42
Average	13-21	24-30	23-30	29-35	30-37
Low	6-12	18-23	18-22	24-28	25-29
Very low	1-5	1-17	1-17	1-23	1-24

Table 4.2: Frequency Distribution of Five Factors of Personality (N=120)

Level of Personality	Number of respondents in different categories									
	N	%	E	%	O	%	A	%	C	%
Very high	54	45	29	24.16	3	2.5	0	0	0	0
High	33	27.5	17	14.16	11	9.16	21	17.5	6	5
Normal	32	26.6	47	39.16	41	34.16	18	15	36	30
Low	1	0.83	10	8.33	41	34.16	52	43.33	15	12.5
Very Low	0	0	17	14.16	24	20	29	24.16	63	52.5

N* Neuroticism, E*Extraversion, O*Openness, A*Agreeableness, C*Conscientiousness

The table 4.2 presents the number of persons falling in five categories from very high to very low for the total sample of 120 respondents. Some of the main observations from the data are as follows.

It is observed that 72.5% of the respondents are falling in either very high or high category on the level of neuroticism whereas only 26.6% respondents are falling in the normal category on Neuroticism. It shows that almost three fourth of the respondents exhibit high or very high neuroticism. High level of neuroticism is related with signs such as emotional reactivity, the tendency to get easily upset and irritated.

Such people are more prone to irrational ideas, and are less able to control their impulses and cope more poorly than others with stressful situations. These people also exhibit sub-traits such as anger, anxiety, self consciousness and vulnerability.

Among the total respondents, 77% have very high to high to normal levels of extraversion. These people enjoy working with people, are more outgoing. The respondents who are average on Extraversion, they are moderate in activity and enthusiasm. They enjoy the company of others but they also value privacy. Remaining 23% respondents have very low to low levels of extraversion. Such people are quiet and do not need any external stimulation to seek energy.

65% of the respondents have scored either very low or low on the Openness to Experience dimension of Big-five personality traits. Open to Experience includes active imagination, preference for variety of things and the readiness for intellectual curiosity and to prefer new experience than routine or familiar way of doing things. It means that 65% of the respondents have not shown these qualities. Only 11% of the respondents are high on Openness. 34% have scored average on this dimension. The persons who are average on Openness have quality of balancing between the old and the new. They are practical but willing to consider new ways of doing things.

From the total sample, 67.49% of respondents are low on Agreeableness. Low agreeableness is related with lack of the traits such as being cooperative and empathetic. Such people are more stubborn, skeptical, proud and competitive than others.

On the level of Conscientiousness, 65% of the respondents have scored very low to low. It shows that such people lack self discipline when it comes to planning and organizing their work. They also show traits such as irresponsibility and are not very well organized. Only 5% have shown high conscientiousness which is associated with the traits such as working diligently for the goals.

Tables 4.3 and 4.4 have presented the frequency distribution for five factors of personality for Non-dance trainees and Dance trainees groups as well.

Table 4.3: Five Factors of Personality for Non-Dance Trainees

(N=60)

Level of Personality	Number of Males (30)										Number of Females (30)									
	N	%	E	%	O	%	A	%	C	%	N	%	E	%	O	%	A	%	C	%
Very High	13	43.3	3	10	1	3.3	0	0	0	0	10	33.3	5	16.6	0	0	0	0	0	
High	7	23.3	3	10	3	10	2	6.6	2	6.66	13	43.3	5	16.6	5	16.6	7	23.3	3	10
Normal	10	33.3	11	36.6	10	33.3	5	16.5	10	33.3	7	23.3	15	50	10	33.3	6	20	8	26.6
Low	0	0	5	16.6	9	30	13	43.3	4	13.3	0	0	1	3.33	9	30	12	40	5	16.6
Very Low	0	0	8	26.6	7	23.3	10	33.3	14	46.6	0	0	4	13.3	6	20	5	16.6	14	46.6

N* Neuroticism, E*Extraversion, O*Openness, A*Agreeableness, C*Conscientiousness

The table 4.3 shows that from 30 male non dance trainees have 43.3% very high neuroticism level it means they are less able to control their impulses and they are very poor to cope up with their stress. They are more emotionally unstable in compare to those who got fewer score on Neuroticism. The table shows that from 30 male non dance trainees 20% respondents are very high on extraversion, 36.6% are having normal, 16.6% have low and 26.6% are having very low on extraversion level.

Some as, from 30 non male dance trainees 3.3% have very high openness level, 10% are high on openness level, 33.3% are having normal, 30% have low and 23.3% are very low on openness level. From some male categories 6.6% are high on Agreeableness, 16.5% are normal, 43.3% are low and 33.3% are very low on Agreeableness. Further, 6.66% are high on conscientiousness, 33.3% are normal, 13.3% are low and 46.6% are very low on conscientiousness. The table is also showing percentage level of female non-dance trainees (30). They are, from 30 non female dance trainees 33.3% are very high on neuroticism, 43.3% are high, 23.3% are normal on Neuroticism. Again from 30 non-dance female trainees 16.6% are very high on Extraversion, 16.6% are high, 50% are normal, 3.33% are low and 13.3% are very low on Extraversion. Some from these female non-dance trainees 16.6% are high on openness, 33.3% are normal, 30% are low and 20% are very low on openness. 23.3% are high on agreeableness, 20% are normal, 40% are low and 16.6% are very low on agreeableness. Among some females 10% are high on conscientiousness, 26.6% are normal, 16.6% are low and 46.6% are very low on conscientiousness.

Table 4.4: Five Factors of Personality for Dance Trainees (N=60)

Level of Personality	Number of Males (30)										Number of Females (30)									
	N	%	E	%	O	%	A	%	C	%	N	%	E	%	O	%	A	%	C	%
Very High	23	76.6	14	46.6	2	6.66	0	0	0	0	8	26.66	7	23.33	0	0	0	0	0	0
High	2	6.66	4	13.3	3	10	4	13.3	0	0	11	36.66	5	26.66	0	0	8	26.6	1	3.33
Normal	5	16.6	8	26.6	9	30	4	13.3	10	33.3	10	33.33	13	43.33	12	40	3	10	8	26.66
Low	0	0	1	3.33	12	40	16	53.3	4	13.33	1	3.33	3	10	11	36.6	11	36.6	2	6.66
Very Low	0	0	3	10	4	13.33	6	20	16	53.33	0	0	2	6.66	7	23.3	8	26.6	19	63.33

N* Neuroticism, E*Extraversion, O*Openness, A*Agreeableness, C*Conscientiousness

The table 4.4 shows that from 30 male dance trainees 76.6% have very high Neuroticism. 46.6% male Dance Trainee respondents are very high on Extraversion. They are more extraverted, outgoing, active and high-spirited respondents.

Further, from 30 female dance trainees only 26.66% are very high on Neuroticism, 36.66% are high, 33.33% are normal and 3.33% are low. Here we can say, from 30 male dance trainees 76.6% are very high on Neuroticism but from 30 female dance trainees there are only 26.66% are very high on Neuroticism. From the same 30 female dance trainees 23.33% are very high on Extraversion, 26.66% are high, 43.33% are normal, 10% are low and 6.66% are very low. 40% are normal on openness, 36.6% are low and 23.3% are very low. Further, from the same female group 26.6% are high on Agreeableness, 10% are normal, 36.6% are low and 26.6% are very low. For conscientiousness, 3.33% females are having high conscientiousness level, 26.66% are normal, 6.66% are low and 63.33% are very low.

4.2.1.2 Mean and Standard Deviation: Personality

The mean, standard deviations and Analysis of Variance for the following five factors of personality have been presented and discussed separately.

- Neuroticism
- Extraversion
- Agreeableness
- Openness
- Conscientiousness

Neuroticism

- As discussed in the previous section based on the frequency distribution, most of the respondents among total sample are Neurotic. They often feel helpless and want someone else to solve their problems. When things go wrong, they get discouraged and feel like giving up. However, it is important to understand the group differences on the level of neuroticism. The table 4.5 shows that the mean Neuroticism score of Dance Trainee female respondents is less than the mean Neuroticism of Non-Dance Trainee male respondents.

- The mean of Dance Trainee male respondents is higher than the mean of Non-Dance Trainee male respondents. It is surprising to note that the non-dancers have less neuroticism than dancers. Although this is due to the highest mean obtained for male dancers group which is 34.2 in comparison to 26.4 for male non-dancers. Among the four groups, male dancers have shown highest level of neuroticism.
- On the other hand, Female dancers have low neuroticism than female non-dancers; it shows that for female, dance training is helpful for low neuroticism.
- Male respondents are more neurotic than female respondents. The mean of Dance Trainee male respondents is higher than the mean of Dance Trainee female respondents. Female respondents are more emotionally stable than male respondents.

Table 4.5: Personality (Neuroticism) - Mean and SD

Gender	Trainee	Mean	Standard Deviation	N
Male	Non- Dance	26.46	7.28	30
	Dance	34.2	8.69	30
	Total	**30.33**	**8.85**	**60**
Female	Non- Dance	26.36	8.06	30
	Dance	23.53	8.64	30
	Total	**24.95**	**8.41**	**60**
Total	**Non- Dance**	**26.41**	**7.61**	**60**
	Dance	**28.86**	**10.14**	**60**
	Total	**27.64**	**8.60**	**120**

Graph 4.1 : Personality (Neuroticism) - Mean

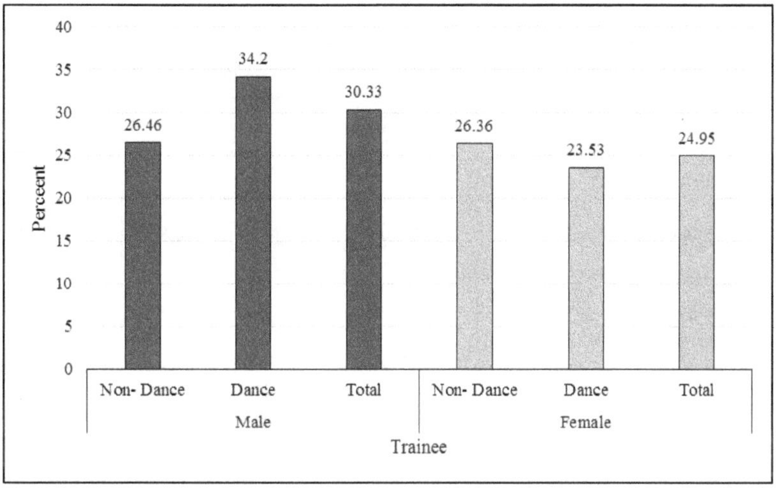

Analysis of Variance: Personality (Neuroticism)

The main aim of Analysis of Variance is to understand whether the means of different groups are statistically significant or not. In this research, a 2x2 factorial design has been used which permits for using a two-way factorial analysis of variance. The two independent variables are Dance Training (Dance Training and Non-Dance Training) and Gender (Male and Female).

The main effect of gender on Neuroticism was found significant at .01 levels. There was a significant effect of Gender on Neuroticism at $F=12.95$, $p<0.01$, there was significantly higher mean score of male (Mean=30.33, sd=8.858) than the mean score of female (mean=24.95, sd=8.412) on Neuroticism. It shows adolescents male have more negative feelings like fear, sadness, embarrassment, guilt, anger etc. in compared to female adolescents.

The main effect of dance training on Neuroticism was not found significant at .01 levels. There is no significantly effect of Dance Training on Neuroticism.

The interaction effect of gender and dance training on the level of neuroticism has been found significant at .01 levels. There was a significant effect of Gender and Dance Training on Neuroticism at $F=12.47$, $p<0.01$.

Table 4.6 - Personality (Neuroticism): Analysis of Variance

ANOVA						
Source of Variation	*Sum of Square*	*df*	*Mean Square*	*F*	*P-value*	*F crit*
Gender (Male & Female)	869.40	1	869.40	12.95	0.00	3.92
Dance Training (Dance trainee & Non-Dance Trainee)	180.07	1	180.07	2.68	0.10	3.92
Interaction effect (Gender * Dance Training	837.40	1	837.40	12.47	0.00	3.90
Within Groups	7786.7	116	67.12			
Total	**9673.59**	**119**				

Extraversion

- The table 4.7 shows that the mean Extraversion of dance trainee male is more than the mean of non-dance trainee male. The male respondents, who were going for any dance training, were more extravert than the male respondents who were not going for any dance training.
- The mean score of Dance Trainee female respondents is more than the mean score of non-dance trainee female respondents.
- For both the male and female respondents, dance Trainee respondents are more extravert in their behavior in comparison to their respective counterparts.
- On the basis of gender, the mean scores of extraversion are 28.16 and 28.7 respectively for male and female respondents. It shows that these groups do not differ on the level of extraversion. It would further be discussed with ANOVA results.
- Among the four groups, the male dancers group has shown higher level of extraversion whereas the male non-dancers group has shown lowest level of extraversion. The mean of Dance Trainee male respondents is more than the mean of Dance Trainee female respondents. It shows the male Dance Trainee respondents are more extravert than the female dance trainee respondents.

Table 4.7: Personality (Extraversion) - Mean and SD

Gender	Trainee	Mean	Standard Deviation	N
Male	Non- Dance	24.16	8.16	30
	Dance	32.16	9.22	30
	Total	28.16	9.47	60
Female	Non- Dance	28.06	7.88	30
	Dance	29.33	7.88	30
	Total	28.7	7.63	60
Total	**Non- Dance**	**26.11**	**8.13**	**60**
	Dance	**30.75**	**8.49**	**60**
	Total	**20.27**	**8.60**	**120**

Graph 4.2: Personality (Extraversion) - Mean

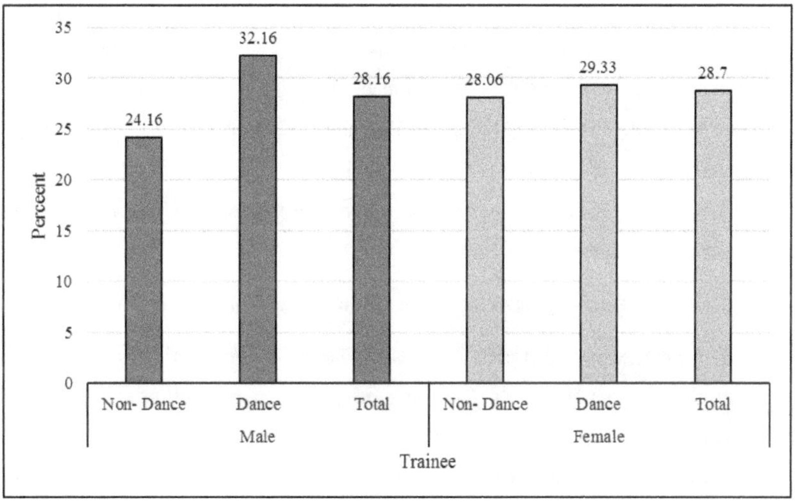

Table 4.8 Personality (Extraversion): Analysis of Variance

ANOVA						
Source of Variation	*Sum of Square*	*df*	*Mean Square*	*F*	*P-value*	*F crit*
Gender (Male & Female)	8.53	1	8.53	0.12	0.72	3.92
Dance Training (Dance trainee & Non-Dance Trainee)	644.03	1	644.03	9.55	0.00	3.92
Interaction effect (Gender * Dance Training)	340.03	1	340.03	5.04	0.02	3.92
Within Groups	7816.86	116	67.38			
Total	**8809.46**	**119**				

The main effect of Dance Training on Extraversion was found significant at 0.01 levels. The dance trainees exhibited more Extraversion than the non-dance trainees. There was a significant effect of Dance Training on Extraversion at $F=9.55$, $p<0.01$, there was significantly higher mean score of Extraversions on dance trainee respondents ($M=30.75$, S.D. = 8.49) than the mean score of Non-Dance Trainee. ($M=26.12$, S.D. = 8.13). Dance Training has significantly affected extraversion. Dancing is a great path to make new friends. It is good social environment where one can easily express his feelings.

The main effect of gender on Extraversion was not found significant.

The interaction effect of Gender and Dance Training on Extraversion was found significant at 0.05 levels There was a significant interaction effect of Gender and Dance Training on Extraversion at $F=5.04$, $p<0.05$. It shows that gender is interacting with dance training to influence extraversion. When the male respondents involve in dance training, their extraversion levels would be higher in comparison to female involved in dance training.

Openness to Experience

- The table 4.9 shows that the Mean Openness score of various groups do not differ much and are close to the overall group (N=120) mean 22.32.
- Table 4.10 shows that the main effect of Dance Training on Openness was not found significant. There is no effect of Dance Training on Openness. Similarly, the main effect of Gender on Openness was also not found significant. There is no effect of gender on Openness. The interaction effect of gender and dance training on openness is also not found significant.

Table 4.9: Personality (Openness) - Mean and SD

Gender	Trainee	Mean	Standard Deviation	N
Male	Non- Dance	22.9	6.25	30
	Dance	22.83	5.97	30
	Total	**22.86**	**6.06**	**60**
Female	Non- Dance	23.43	6.40	30
	Dance	20.13	3.69	30
	Total	**21.78**	**5.44**	**60**
Total	**Non- Dance**	**23.16**	**6.28**	**60**
	Dance	**21.48**	**5.10**	**60**
	Total	**22.32**	**5.76**	**120**

Graph 4.3: Personality (Openness) - Mean

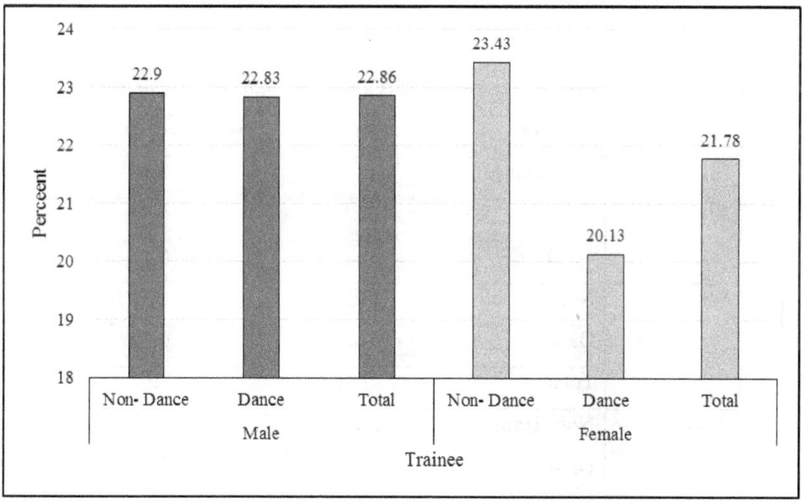

Table 4.10 Personality (Openness): Analysis of Variance

ANOVA						
Source of Variation	*Sum of Square*	*df*	*Mean Square*	*F*	*P-value*	*F crit*
Gender (Male & Female)	35.20	1	35.20	1.08	0.29	3.92
Dance Training (Dance trainee & Non-Dance Trainee)	85.00	1	85.00	2.62	0.10	3.92
Interaction effect (Gender * Dance Training	78.40	1	78.40	2.42	0.12	3.92
Within Groups	3755.7	116	32.37			
Total	**3954.32**	**119**				

Agreeableness

- The table 4.11 shows that the Mean Agreeableness score of various groups do not differ much and are close to the overall group (N=120) mean 26.35.
- Table 4.12 shows that the main effect of Dance Training on Agreeableness was not found significant. There is no effect of Dance Training on Agreeableness. Similarly, the main effect of Gender on Agreeableness was also not found significant. There is no effect of gender on Agreeableness. The interaction effect of gender and dance training on Agreeableness is also not found significant.

Table 4.11: Personality (Agreeableness) - Mean and SD

Gender	Trainee	Mean	Standard deviation	N
Male	Non- Dance	24.7	5.34	30
	Dance	25.8	6.80	30
	Total	25.25	6.11	60
Female	Non- Dance	28.16	6.99	30
	Dance	26.73	6.99	30
	Total	27.45	7.62	60
Total	**Non- Dance**	**26.43**	**6.41**	**60**
	Dance	**26.26**	**7.53**	**60**
	Total	**26.35**	**6.96**	**120**

Graph 4.4: Personality (Agreeableness) - Mean

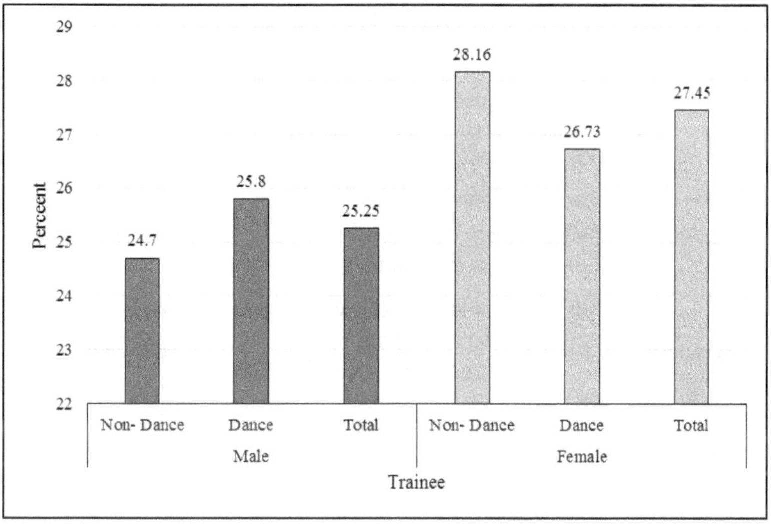

Table 4.12 Personality (Agreeableness): Analysis of Variance

ANOVA						
Source of Variation	*Sum of Square*	*df*	*Mean Square*	*F*	*P-value*	*F crit*
Gender (Male & Female)	145.2	1	145.2	3.01	0.08	3.92
Dance Training (Dance trainee & Non-Dance Trainee)	0.83	1	0.83	0.01	0.89	3.92
Interaction effect (Gender * Dance Training	48.13	1	48.13	0.99	0.31	3.92
Within Groups	5585.13	116	48.14			
Total	**5779.3**	**119**				

Conscientiousness

- The table 4.13 shows that the Mean Agreeableness score of various groups do not differ much and are close to the overall group (N=120) mean 26.63.
- Table 4.14 shows that the main effect of Dance Training on Conscientiousness was not found significant. There is no effect of Dance Training on Conscientiousness. Similarly, the main effect of Gender on Conscientiousness was also not found significant. There is no effect of gender on Conscientiousness. The interaction effect of gender and dance training on Conscientiousness is also not found significant.

Table 4.13: Personality (Conscientiousness) - Mean and SD

Gender	Trainee	Mean	Standard Deviation	N
Male	Non- Dance	26.76	7.16	30
	Dance	27	6.00	30
	Total	26.88	6.55	60
Female	Non- Dance	26.96	6.77	30
	Dance	25.8	7.5	30
	Total	26.38	7.12	60
Total	**Non- Dance**	**26.86**	**6.91**	**60**
	Dance	**26.4**	**6.77**	**60**
	Total	**26.63**	**6.82**	**120**

Graph 4.5: Personality (Conscientiousness) - Mean

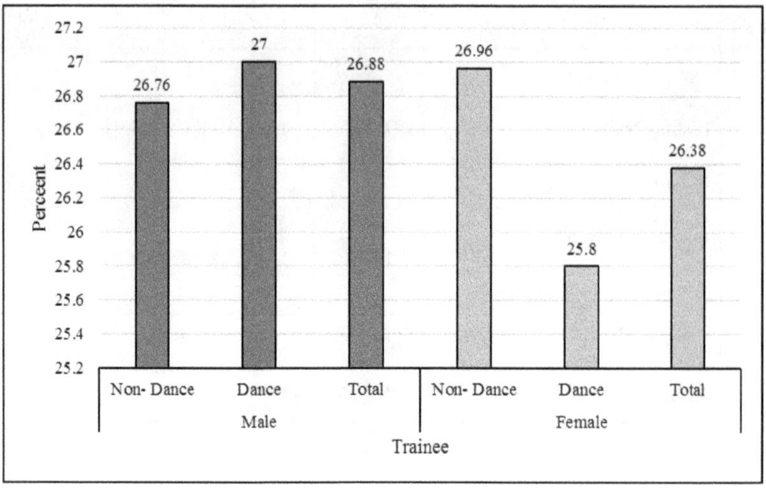

Table 4.14 Personality (Conscientiousness): Analysis of Variance

ANOVA						
Source of Variation	*Sum of Square*	*df*	*Mean Square*	*F*	*P-value*	*F crit*
Gender (Male & Female)	7.5	1	7.5	0.15	0.69	3.92
Dance Training (Dance trainee & Non-Dance Trainee)	6.53	1	6.53	0.13	0.71	3.92
Interaction effect (Gender * Dance Training	14.7	1	14.7	0.30	0.57	3.92
Within Groups	5507.13	116	47.47			
Total	**5535.66**	**119**				

4.2.2 Anxiety

4.2.2.1 Frequency Distribution

Table 4.15: Level of anxiety for the total sample (N=120)

Level of Anxiety	Number of respondents (N=120)	Percentage
Very high	0	0
High	11	9.16
Normal	56	46.66
Low	34	28.33
Very low	19	15.83

The table 4.12 shows that 46.66% have normal anxiety, 28.33% low anxiety, 15.83 % very low anxiety and 9.16% are having very high anxiety level.

Table 4.16: Levels of Anxiety for the Non-Dance Trainee Group (N=60)

Level of Anxiety	Number of males (N=30)	Percentage	Number of females (N=30)	Percentage	Total respondents (n=60)	Percentage
Very high	0	0	0	0	0	0
High	5	16.66	6	20	11	18.33
Normal	12	40	12	40	24	40
Low	10	33.33	9	30	19	31.66
Very low	3	10	3	10	6	10

Table 4.17: Levels of Anxiety for the Dance Trainees Group (N=60)

Level of Anxiety	Number of males (N=30)	Percentage (%)	Number of females (N=30)	Percentage	Total respondents (n=60)	Percentage (%)
Very high	0	0	0	0	0	0
High	0	0	0	0	0	0
Normal	18	60	14	46.66	32	53.33
Low	6	20	9	30	15	25
Very low	6	20	7	23.33	13	21.66

4.2.2.3 Mean and Standard Deviation: Anxiety

- The table 4.18 shows the mean Anxiety score of Dance Trainee group is less than the mean of Non-Dance Trainee group. It shows Dance Training group has less anxiety.
- The Dance Trainee respondents are more optimistic than Non-Dance Trainee respondents. They can sleep easily without any tension. They are mentally stronger than Non-Dance Trainee respondents. They never worried about small things. They believe in positivity more than Non-Dance Trainee respondents.
- The female respondents have more Anxiety than male respondents, however, this difference is not found to be statistically significant.

Table 4.18: Mean and Standard Deviation - Anxiety

Gender	Trainee	Mean	Standard Deviation	N
Male	Non- Dance	25.7	7.40	30
	Dance	22.73	5.80	30
	Total	24.21	6.76	60
Female	Non- Dance	28.53	9.09	30
	Dance	22.5	4.89	30
	Total	25.51	7.85	60
Total	**Non- Dance**	**27.11**	**8.34**	**60**
	Dance	**22.61**	**5.32**	**60**
	Total	**20.27**	**8.08**	**120**

Table 4.6: Anxiety – Mean

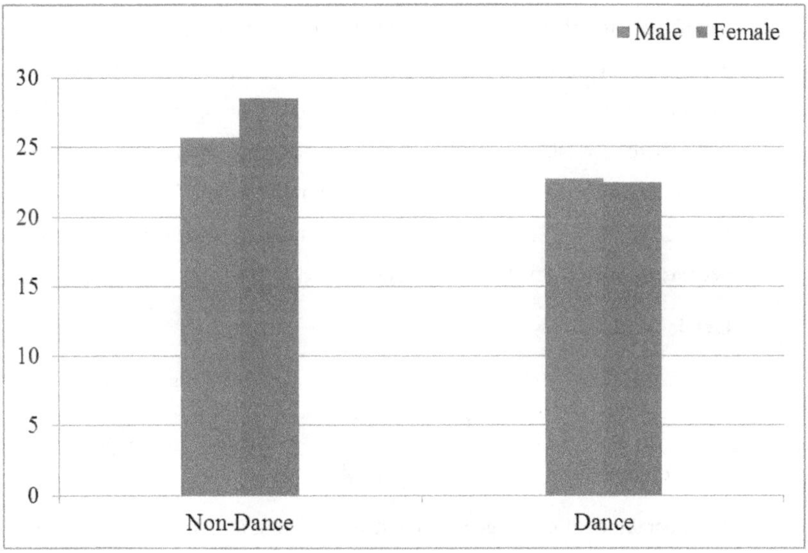

4.2.2.4 Analysis of Variance: Anxiety

Table 4.19 Analysis of Variance - Anxiety

ANOVA						
Source of Variation	***Sum of Square***	***df***	***Mean Square***	***F***	***P-value***	***F crit***
Gender (Male & Female)	50.7	1	50.7	1.0385	0.31029	3.922
Dance Training (Dance trainee & Non-Dance Trainee)	607.5	1	607.5	12.443	0.000602	3.922
Interaction effect (Gender * Dance Training	70.533	1	70.533	1.444	0.231819	3.922
Within Groups	5663.133	116	48.820			
Total	**6391.866**	**119**				

Dance Training and Anxiety

Table 4.20 shows that the main effect of dance training on anxiety was found significant at .01 levels. The respondents who were undergoing dance training, experienced less anxiety as compared to those who were not taking any dance training. There was a significant effect of dance training on anxiety at F= 12.44, p< .000, there was significantly higher mean score of anxiety on non-dance trainee respondents (M= 27.11, S.D. 8.34) than the mean score of dance trainee respondents (M= 22.61, S.D.= 5.32). The result concluded that dance training is good for decreasing anxiety level in respondents.

Gender and Anxiety:

The main effect of Gender on Anxiety was not found significant. There was non-significant effect of Gender on Anxiety at F=1.03, p=0.31.

Interaction Effect:

The interaction effect of gender and dance training on Anxiety was also not found to be significant. There is no difference in the level of Anxiety among male and female who were going for dance training. There was non-significant interaction effect of Gender and dance training on Anxiety at F=1.444, p=0.23.

4.2.3 Psychophysical Health

4.2.3.1 Mean and Standard Deviation: Psychophysical Health

Physical Health

- The table 4.21 shows mean Physical health of Dance Trainee respondents is less than the mean of Non-Dance Trainee respondents. The less the score is, the better the Physical health is.
- The Dance Trainee respondents have better physical health than the Non-Dance Trainee respondents. Dance is best exercise for our body. Respondents become more flexible and fit through Dance. Dance Training increased muscular strength, improve posture and flexibility. It is also helpful in reduce pain and stiffness.
- The female respondents have better Physical health than the male respondents.
- Male Dance Trainee respondents are more physically fit than female Dance Trainee respondents. Male Dance Trainee respondents feel less Dizziness than others. They are not much worried about their health. They are less suffering from headache and other physical health related problems than their comparison group.
- Among the four groups, male dance trainee groups showed best physical health whereas male non-dancers suffered the most with physical health related issues.

Table 4.20: Mean and Standard Deviation: Physical Health

Gender	Trainee	Mean	Standard Deviation	N
Male	Non- Dance	7.43	2.35	30
	Dance	0.86	0.93	30
	Total	4.15	3.75	60
Female	Non- Dance	5.33	1.34	30
	Dance	1.43	1.50	30
	Total	3.38	2.42	60
Total	**Non- Dance**	**6.38**	**2.17**	**60**
	Dance	**1.15**	**1.27**	**60**
	Total	**3.76**	**3.17**	**120**

Graph 4.7: Physical Health – Mean

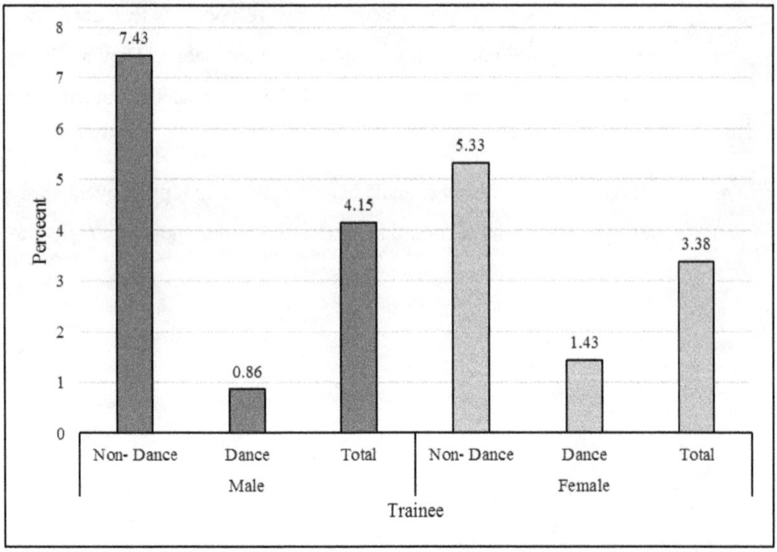

Table 4.21 Analysis of Variance: Physical Health

ANOVA						
Source of Variation	*Sum of Square*	*df*	*Mean Square*	*F*	*P-value*	*F crit*
Gender (Male & Female)	821.63	1	821.63	312.62	.000	3.92
Dance Training (Dance trainee & Non-Dance Trainee)	17.63	1	17.63	6.70	0.025	3.92
Interaction effect (Gender * Dance Training	53.33	1	53.33	20.29	.000	3.92
Within Groups	304.86	116	2.62			
Total	**1197.46**	**119**				

The main effect of Dance training on Physical health was found significant at 0.01 levels. There was a significant effect of Dance training on Physical health at F=6.70, p=0.01, there was significantly higher mean score of non-dance trainees (Mean=6.38, S.D. =2.17) than the mean score of dance trainees (mean=1.15, S.D.=1.27) on Physical health.

The main effect of Gender on Physical health was found significant at 0.01 levels. There was a significant effect of Gender on Physical health at F=312.62, p<0.00, there was significantly higher mean score of male respondents (Mean=4.15, S.D. =3.75) than the mean score of female (mean=3.35, S.D.=2.42) on Physical health. The interaction effect of Gender and Dance Training on Physical health was also found significant at 0.01 levels.

Mental Health

- The table 4.22 shows Dance Trainee respondents have good mental health than Non-Dance Trainee respondents. The Dance Trainee respondents can easily adjust in any situation than others. They are able to handle every situation with positivity. They have more control on their emotions in compare to Non-Dance Trainee respondents. Similarly, female respondents have better mental health the male respondents. Among the four groups, the male dance trainee groups showed the best mental health whereas the male non-dance trainee group suffered the most with mental health related issues.

- Table 4.23 shows that the main effect of Dance training on Mental health was found significant at 0.01 levels. There was a significant effect of Dance training on Mental health at $F=338.77$, $p<0.000$, there was significantly higher mean score of non-dance trainees (Mean=8.03, S.D. =3.61) than the mean score of dance trainees (mean=1.2, S.D.=1.05) on Mental health.
- Table 4.23 also shows that the main effect of Gender on Mental health was found significant at 0.01 levels. There was a significant effect of Gender on Mental health at $F=6.70$, $p<0.05$, there was significantly higher mean score of male respondents (Mean=5.78, S.D. =5.29) than the mean score of female (mean=3.45, S.D.=2.66) on Mental health. The interaction effect of Gender and Dance Training on Mental health was also found significant at 0.01 levels.

Table 4.22: Mean and Standard Deviation- Mental Health

Gender	Trainee	Mean	Standard Deviation	N
Male	Non- Dance	10.46	3.61	30
	Dance	1.1	0.84	30
	Total	5.78	5.29	60
Female	Non- Dance	5.6	1.83	30
	Dance	1.3	1.2	30
	Total	3.45	2.66	60
Total	**Non- Dance**	**8.03**	**3.61**	**60**
	Dance	**1.2**	**1.05**	**60**
	Total	**8.03**	**4.33**	**120**

Graph 4.8 : Mental Health – Mean

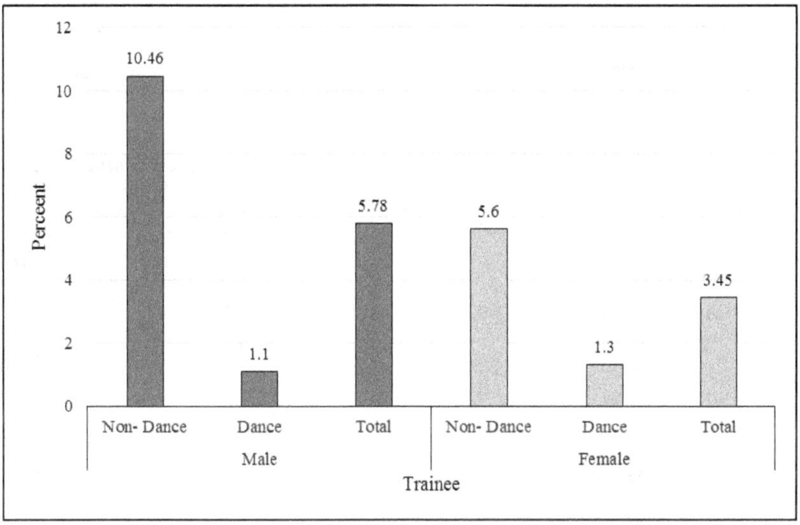

Table 4.23 Analysis of Variance - Mental Health

ANOVA						
Source of Variation	*Sum of Square*	*df*	*Mean Square*	*F*	*P-value*	*F crit*
Gender (Male & Female)	163.33	1	163.33	39.49	.000	3.92
Dance Training (Dance trainee & Non-Dance Trainee)	1400.83	1	1400.83	338.77	.000	3.92
Interaction effect (Gender * Dance Training	192.53	1	192.53	46.56	.000	3.92
Within Groups	479.66	116	4.13			
Total	**2236.36**	**119**				

Psychophysical Health

This section presents results for Psychophysical health which represents the overall health scores obtained from the total scores of Area A i.e. Physical health and Area B i.e. Mental Health.

Table 4.24: Mean and Standard deviation: Dance Training and Psychophysical Health

	N	Mean	Deviation	Std. Error	df	p. Value
Dance Trainee	60	2.35	2.073	0.268		
Non-Dance Trainee	60	14.40	5.228	0.675	118	0.000

Graph 4.9 : Dance Training and Psychophysical Health - Mean

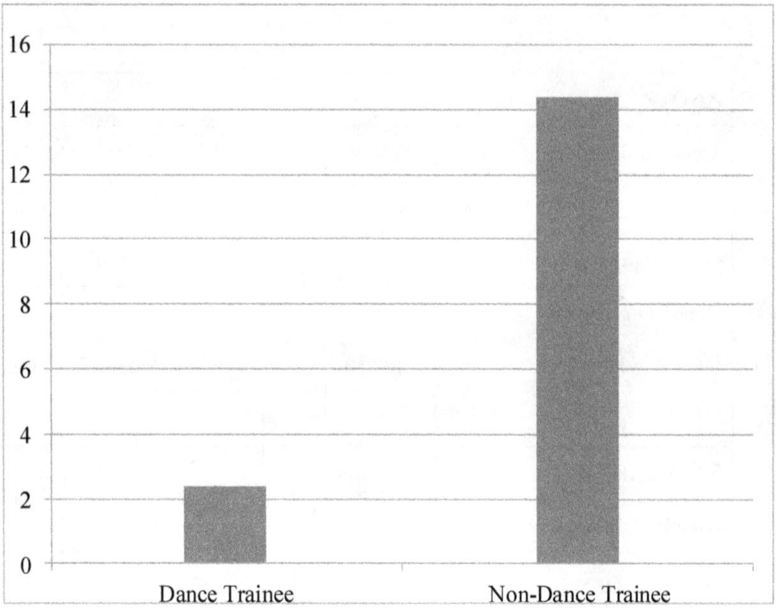

- Table 4.24 shows the Psychophysical Health of Dance Trainee respondents is better in comparison to the Non-Dance Trainee respondents.

Table 4.25: Mean and Standard Deviation: Gender and Psychophysical Health

	N	Mean	Deviation	Std. Error	df	p. Value
Male	60	10.30	8.504	1.098		
Female	60	6.45	5.060	0.653	118	0.003

Graph 4.10: Gender and Psychophysical Health - Mean

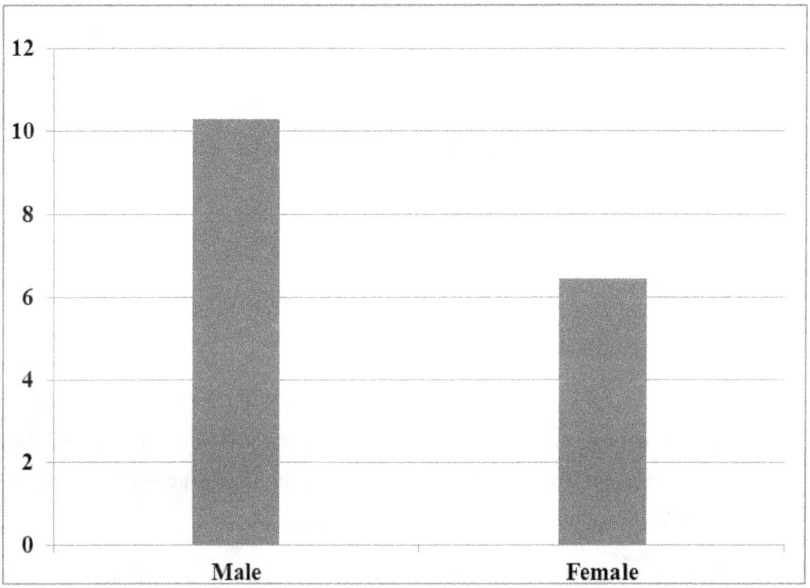

- The table 4.25 shows Gender and P.G.I. total Psychophysical health scores. The mean of male respondents is 10.30 and the mean of female respondents is 6.45. The mean of female is less than the mean of male respondents. The female respondents are more physically and mentally fit in comparison to male respondents.

4.2.3.2 Analysis of Variance: Psychophysical Health

The main effect of dance training of Psychophysical health was found significant at 0.01 levels. The respondents, who were going for dance training, were physically and mentally health as compared to those who were not taking any dance training. There was a significant effect of dance training on Psychophysical health at F=257.96, P<0.000, the result concluded that dance training is good for physical health of respondents. The respondents, who were going for dance training, were mentally health as compared to those who were not taking any dance training. Constant movements during dance results into improve cardiovascular functioning. During dance the heart beat as faster as, fast dance is done which makes heart strong and healthier. Lower body strength and overall core strength can be improving with the help of dance as it requires fancy footwork which is excellent for legs and core strength. Dance has positive impact on the mind too. Moving on favorite song, gives us happiness, and we are able to reconnect with over selves. The main effect of Gender on Psychophysical health was found significant at 0.05 levels. The result concluded that female respondents are more physically and mentally health in compared to male respondents. The interaction effect of Gender and Dance Training on Psychophysical Health was not found to be significant.

Phase-II

Intervention Phase: Dance Movement Therapy

In the second phase, 20 persons were selected from the Non-dance trainees' group and were randomly assigned to two groups; each group included 10 persons. It was also randomly decided which group would receive the treatment; hence control group and experimental group were also randomly decided.

Pre-testing data for all the three dependent variables was already available from Phase-I. Post-testing data was obtained after the intervention model implemented on the experimental group. The experimental group was provided dance-movement therapy sessions for four weeks by using the techniques mentioned in the proposed intervention model prepared by the researcher. The intervention model and its techniques have already been discussed in detail in Chapter-3. The effect of DMT intervention was studied on the Personality, Psychophysical health and the level of Anxiety. The significance of the difference between means of both control and experimental group was studied by using t-test. The results obtained for Phase-II will be discussed now.

Intervention Phase Results

(1) Personality

(a) Neuroticism

Table 4.26: Neuroticism and Dance Movement Therapy

Control Group		Experimental group	
Pretest score	Post test score	Pretest score	Post test score
Mean=23.4	Mean=23.2	Mean=19.9	Mean=17.9
0.79		0.02 Significant	

The effect of dance movement therapy on Neuroticism was found significant at 0.02 levels. There was a significant effect of dance movement therapy on Neuroticism in the experimental group. The difference in the neuroticism levels among the control group did not differ significantly. It can be concluded that the neuroticism level decreased in the experimental group due to the intervention in the form of dance movement therapy. The result shows dance movement Therapy effect Neuroticism. Neuroticism includes feeling of fear, jealousy, guilt, anger, worry, frustration and loneliness etc. It is possible to manage these negative feelings through dance movement therapy.

(b) Extraversion

Table 4.27: Extraversion and Dance Movement Therapy

Control Group		Experimental group	
Pretest score	Post test score	Pretest score	Post test score
Mean=28.9	Mean=26	Mean=24.9	Mean=30.4
0.37		0.00 Significant	

The effect of dance movement therapy on extraversion was found significant at 0.00 levels. There was a significant effect of dance movement therapy on Extraversion. The experimental group which had undergone dance movement therapy sessions reported high levels of extraversion. It indicates dance can help to increase the extraversion. It was seen that the experimental group who had been undergoing dance movement therapy for 3 months, they were easily able to talk to others, and they would quickly mix with others.

(c) Openness

Table 4.28: Openness and Dance Movement Therapy

Control Group		Experimental group	
Pretest score	Post test score	Pretest score	Post test score
Mean=24.1	Mean=24.1	Mean=23.5	Mean=23.5
		Non-significant	

The effect of dance movement therapy on openness was not found significant. There was non-significant effect of dance movement therapy on openness.

(d) Agreeableness

Table 4.29: Agreeableness and Dance Movement Therapy

Control Group		Experimental group	
Pretest score	Post test score	Pretest score	Post test score
Mean=27.8	Mean=27.8	Mean=26	Mean=24.6
		Non-significant	

The effect of dance movement therapy on Agreeableness was not found significant. The dance movement therapy has no effect on tendency of Agreeableness.

(e) Conscientiousness

Table 4.30: Conscientiousness and Dance Movement Therapy

Control Group		Experimental group	
Pretest score	Post test score	Pretest score	Post test score
Mean=28.2	Mean=27.2	Mean=26.6	Mean=26.1
		Non-significant	

The effect of dance movement therapy on conscientiousness was not found significant. The pre-test and post-test mean of experimental groups did not differ significantly.

(2) Anxiety

Table 4.31: Anxiety and Dance Movement Therapy

Control Group		Experimental group	
Pretest score	Post test score	Pretest score	Post test score
Mean=21.6	Mean=17.2	Mean=20.3	Mean=18.2
0.02 Significant		0.02 Significant	

Here, the level of anxiety in both groups is decreasing in post-test, it means the level of anxiety is decreasing but it cannot be concluded that the decrease in the level of anxiety is due to dance movement therapy intervention; because this decrease is also reported in the control group which is also significant.

(3) Psychophysical Health

Table 4.32: Physical Health and Dance Movement Therapy

Control Group		Experimental group	
Pretest score	Post test score	Pretest score	Post test score
Mean=4.4	Mean=3.4	Mean=5.9	Mean=3.9
0.12 Non-significant		0.00 Significant	

The effect of dance movement therapy on Physical Health was found significant at 0.00 levels. There was a significant effect of dance movement therapy on physical health. There was significantly lower mean score of experimental groups post-test (M=3.9) in comparison to the pre-test (M=5.9). Lower scores means better physical health. The mean value of control group (m=3.4) is also decreasing in post-test but this difference in the pre-test and post-test scores of the control group is not significant. It can be concluded that dance movement therapy is helpful in improving physical health. Movements are good for muscles strength, body flexibility and to reduce fat.

Table 4.33: Mental Health and Dance Movement Therapy

Control Group		Experimental group	
Pretest score	Post test score	Pretest score	Post test score
Mean=4.4	Mean=2.6	Mean=10.7	Mean=6.2
0.01 Significant		0.000 Significant	

The mean Mental health scores of both groups are decreasing that means the mental health has shown improvements in both control and experimental groups; hence it cannot be concluded that Dance Movement Therapy has resulted in improvement in mental health. Although the difference in the experimental group is statistically significant at .000 levels in comparison to the control group where the means values differ significantly at .01 levels. The means scores have improved from 10.7 to 6.2 in the experimental group in comparison to the control groups where the mean mental health score have improved from 4.4 to 2.6. It shows that DMT has posed better improvement in the mental health.

On the basis of the above results, the following observations can be drawn.

- Therapeutic Dance is good for decreasing Neuroticism level and increasing Extraversion in behaviour. The different techniques of session help to positively affect these dimensions of the participants' personality. They help to develop social skills as well as the ability to regulate one's emotional reactivity, impulsivity, anger etc.
- Therapeutic Dance is also good to remain physically healthy. Dance is a good exercise. Through dance exercise one can reduce fat and remain healthy and fit. Stretching is good to make body more flexible. Breathing exercise is beneficial to reduce stress. DMT has also found to be effective in improving mental health.

Participants' Experiences about DMT

When researcher asked the participants about their experiences of dancing regularly since last 4 weeks, they said they feel relaxed and they felt more connected to themselves and they didn't want to leave the dance class as long as possible. It gives them instant relief. The respondents who were in the job somewhere, they told the researcher that after office time, when they join dance class daily, they feel refresh, energetic and when they practice 'cool down' in dance session, they feel calm and relaxed. The researcher also talked to some choreographers, Rajasthan, they told that whenever they were anxious, they do practice Dance.

4.3 HYPOTHESIS TESTING:

This section represents Hypothesis testing, in which researcher found through obtained results, whether hypothesis have been accepted or rejected.

1. There is no difference between the personality of dance trainee and non-dance trainee.

- ➢ This null hypothesis has been partially accepted and partially rejected. The difference in extraversion is found to be significantly different between dance trainees and non-dance trainees; but the these groups do not differ significantly on the other four factors Neuroticism, Openness, Agreeableness and Conscientiousness.

2. There is no difference between the psychophysical health of dance training and non-dance training.

- ➢ This hypothesis has been rejected as the mean of dance trainee on psychophysical health is less than the mean of non-dance trainee. The effect of dance training on psychophysical health was found significant at 0.000 levels. There is difference between the psychophysical health of dance trainee and non-dance trainee, where the dance trainees have better psychophysical health than the non-dance trainee group.

3. There is no difference between the level of anxiety of dance trainee and non-dance trainee.

- ➢ This null hypothesis has been rejected as there is difference between the level of anxiety of dance trainee and non-dance trainee. the anxiety of non-dance trainee is more than the level of anxiety among dance trainees. The effect of dance training on Anxiety was found significant at 0.000 levels.

4. There is no difference between the personality of males and females.

➢ This null hypothesis has been partially accepted and partially rejected as there is no difference between the personality of males and females on four of the five factors i.e. extraversion, openness, agreeableness and conscientiousness; however the effect of Gender on Neuroticism was found significant at 0.001 levels.

5. There is no difference between the psychophysical health of males and females.

➢ This null hypothesis has been rejected as the Psychophysical health of female respondents is better than the male respondents. There is difference between the psychophysical health of males and females. The effect of gender on Psychophysical health was found significant at 0.01 levels.

6. There is no difference between the level of anxiety of males and females.

➢ This null hypothesis has been accepted as there is no difference between the level of anxiety of males and females. The effect of gender on anxiety was found non-significant.

7. There is no effect of therapeutic use of dance movement therapy on personality, psychophysical health and anxiety.

This hypothesis is partially accepted and partially rejected. The therapeutic use of dance movement therapy has significantly affected neuroticism and extraversion dimension among the five factors of personality. The other three factors openness, agreeableness and conscientiousness have not been affected significantly by the dance movement therapy intervention. The DMT intervention has also not affected the level of anxiety and mental health. However, the physical health as improved due to the intervention.

4.4 FURTHER DISCUSSION

Dance is a form of physical exercise. An individual involves not only physically in the dancing but the other aspects such as mental, cognitive and affective domains are also involved. This further strengthens an individual's psychomotor aspects. It provides body balance and coordination to the body. When a dancer remembers certain steps and techniques of dancing, it strengthens various cognitive activities such as attention, concentration, memory, thinking etc.

As a form of physical activity, many dance classes organize dance sessions for various other dance forms. It provides flexibility to the body, it leads to better blood circulation, sweating and cleansing of the body fluids. It revitalizes and rejuvenates the body. Cardiovascular benefits of physical exercises are also obtained in the process of dancing. Dance exercise is helpful in strengthening our bones and muscles. Increased level of physical activity can help intercept illness such as diabetes, heart disease and reduce the risk of osteoporosis as bones become stronger. These reasons lead to improvement in the Physical health due to dance.

When an individual engages in dance practice, it poses challenges to the individual's brain. Focusing on certain steps and being able to follow those steps and techniques requires body coordination and cognitions. Recalling the constant changing movement in the desired sequence requires the brain to function faster. The brain works on both sensory and motor functions, cognitive functions which improves the neural circuits in the brain. Dance is, thus the best form of mental exercise also. A study published in the New England Journal of Medicine, suggested that dance can improve brain health. Researchers examined the effect that different 11 types of physical activities on elderly participants. These involved cycling, swimming, tennis and golf. Only dancing lowered the participant's risk of dementia.

Dance is also found to be associated with one's emotions. The facial expressions, body gestures and postures not only help in expressing one's emotions but to be able to generate positive emotions. An individual feels sense of achievement and confidence which further improves the mental health. The dancers become more emotionally intelligent. The present research has also found that dancers are less neurotic than the non-dancers. It means that dancers can better regulate their moods and emotions. Dance also provides an opportunity to ventilate one's feelings in the form of catharsis. It is also said 'letting loose' helps in reducing the level of stress and anxiety also.

Dance can also help in improvement of the interpersonal relationships. As found in the present research also, the people involved in dancing develop more extraversion among them, due to which they interact more with others and are more sociable. The dancers develop betters ways of dealing with others and dealing with their relationships. It improves their social life. When the social aspects are strengthens, it improves the other aspects as well.

Through dance, one can also connect with own body. One can directly express himself through body with the dance being the most fundamental of arts. It can open interesting doorways to our psyche by understanding the relationship with body. Dance includes another important element that is music. The individual listens to the music and to the words/lyrics. All these elements helps in becoming aware of ourselves, our limitations and our movement preferences, our fear of non-verbal expressions degree of confidence in attitude and monotony of moving in conditioned way. All of these factors will impact our relationship with environment and our personality and behavior.

The findings, published in the New England Journal of Medicine suggested that Dancing on a regular basis is associated with a 76 percent reduction in dementia risk. It was said that if an individual does not find exercise to be an enjoyable activity, the person will not get involved in it. Dancing is thus an exercise which involves entertainment, rhythm, music. The enjoyable involvement in dance can trigger the release of feel good hormones like serotonin and endorphins.

Some other research works have supported the findings of the present work. Arpita C. (2013) studied that Dance increases total body movement, which helps to improve circulatory, respiratory, skeletal and muscular systems. It has a positive effect on physical health as well as mental and emotional welling. Mastura J., Mardian S. and Haizan T. (2015) studied the effect of a 12 week low intensity dance exercise intervention in the treatment of hostility subscale, anxiety subscale and depression subscale among overweight women working in Malaysia. The result concluded that the dance intervention had contributed positively to physical health as well as psychological well-being. Kiraly, Urban, Griffiths & Demetrrics studied that dancing is a popular form of physical exercise and studies have shown that dancing can decrease anxiety, increase self-esteem and improve psychological wellbeing.

The dance and therapeutic dance have also been found helpful in controlling various mental ailments be it depression, anxiety, dementia, attention deficit hyperactivity disorder etc.

Sobline, Teresa, Sissy & Roleyn (2014) studied the effect of dance movement therapy on health related psychological problems. Results suggested that dance is effective for increasing quality of life and decreasing clinical symptoms such as depression and anxiety. According to a study published in Frontiers in Human Neuroscience, "dancing may be a better form of exercise than traditional fitness training when it comes to slowing the signs of aging. This is because of the added mental challenges required, which include remembering dance steps. Holding the partner in right way, executing turns, recognizing the beat and synchronizing movement with music, all of these activities are mentioned to as "sensorimotor demands". They relate to bodily activity or movement triggered by sensory as well as motor impulses."

Gronlund, Renck & Weileull (2005) studied a short-term dance movement therapy for two young boys with symptoms related to Attention Deficit Hyperactivity Disorder (ADHD). The DMT has promoted a positive change to a certain extent. DMT provided in paired groups for a minimum of ten weeks will (1) improve the motor function and (2) reduce the behavioural and emotional symptoms of boys with ADHD.

Another study at the University of Illinois at Chicago examined a Latin ballroom dance program for older sedentary adults. The senior dancers disclosed improvements in memory, focus and attention, through the programme. The memory and thinking of participants had improved after the 10-month long dancing session. The same study concluded that "Age related degeneration in brain structure and cognitive impairment may be mitigated with physical activity, especially dance. This is because dance requires more than just motor skills so there is more thinking associated with it."

Conclusion

In the present research, dance has been beneficial for neuroticism factor of personality, physical health, mental health and level of anxiety. The other personality factors such as extraversion, agreeableness, openness to experience and conscientiousness have not been found to be affected by dance movement therapy. The minimum duration dance training was kept three months as the inclusion criteria in the present research. The average dance training duration for the 60 dance trainees in the dance trainee (DT) group was 5 months. One reason for not getting significant result may be the duration of dance training. The dance training might have long term effect on some other variables. The average 5-month training duration might not be sufficient for the dance to show its positive effects on the psychological aspects of an individual. The dance training duration can be increased in further researches to get a better picture of dance training.

The Dance Movement Therapy intervention was also planned for 4 weeks. DMT has also shown positive effect on extraversion also which was not significant with the dance training. It is recommended for further researches to plan dance-movement therapy sessions for longer duration than four-weeks for getting better results.

Dance has been found to be having benefits on the physical and mental health. It also lowers level of neuroticism. It also helps in lowering the level of anxiety. The dance movement therapy can have positive effect on making individual more extraverted, excitement seeking, gregarious, assertive and motives them to involve more with the external world.

CHAPTER-5

IMPLICATIONS, SUGGESTIONS AND LIMITATIONS

The outcomes of a research must be understood and the knowledge obtained through the findings should subsequently be used for the benefit of the society at large. This chapter presents some implications based on the present research findings. Implications refer to how the findings of a particular research can be important for practitioners, policy decision makers, for theory builders of a discipline and for the future researchers. This chapter has also listed certain suggestions for the future researchers which will be useful in framing research objectives, selecting relevant variables and methodology for further researches. No research can be free from any limitations due to constraints of the time, available funds and the manpower. Some limitations of this research are also discussed in this chapter.

The present research has studied the effect of dance training and gender on personality, psychophysical health and anxiety. It has been found that dance affects certain dimensions of personality, anxiety and psychophysical health of an individual. The effect of Dance Movement Therapy as an intervention has also been studied and found to be effective. The use of various arts forms as therapeutic interventions are being used. The use of dance as a form of physical exercise, recreational activity and as a psychotherapeutic alternative is recommended for the treatment of various mental health issues.

5.1 IMPLICATIONS

Certain benefits of dance and dance movement therapy have been discussed along with the implications of this research for the benefit of the society.

- **Promotion of Dance Movement Therapy:** On the basis of the findings of the present research, there is a need to increase the use of Dance Movement Therapy as a part of psychotherapeutic intervention. Looking at the demographic profile at global and national level, it has been found that youth have suffered from the issues of anxiety and other related mental health issues. It is recommended that the psychotherapists, psychologists, mental health practitioners can be trained on the use of Dance Movement Therapy so that skilled dance movement therapist can be available to use dance movement therapy as a therapeutic intervention to control the level of anxiety, stress and depression among the general population.

- **Skilled and Competent DMT Professionals:** Availability of trained professions who can use dance as a form of psychotherapy is also a challenge. More training workshops are needed for preparing a pool of competent and skilled DMT professionals. The training programs need to be supported by allocating funds through various governmental schemes to make these workshops affordable to the aspiring DMT professionals.

- **Inclusion in Personality Development Programmes:** Dance training also helps in improving some personality dimensions such as extraversion and neuroticism among adolescents. Dance Training as a form of physical exercise can be a part of personality development programmes. In this research it is found that dance is helpful in enhancing extrovert behaviour of individual which means the one who practices dance on regular basis makes an individual more expressive, assertive who can communication oneself with others which leads to increase in confidence level in the person.

- **Budget in Health Policy:** There is a need to promote use of various art therapies in clinical settings. Sufficient budget need to be allocated to the institutes and professionals who provide various forms of art therapy including dance training and dance movement therapy. Health policy makers must include dance which is a form of physical exercises which not only affects physical health related parameters but it also helps in improving emotions, moods, personality and also contributes positively at the interpersonal relationship fronts.

- **Mental Health Issues:** It has been established in the present and many other researches that dance helps in reducing anxiety level. Researchers have shown that when we perform dance our body releases endorphins and this hormone reduces depression, anxiety and stress. In day to day life most of the people suffer with anxiety and related symptoms. There are many reasons behind increase in anxiety level such as stress at work, stress from school, financial stress, stress in personal life for example stress in marriage, stress from an emotional trauma like death of loved one, stress from serious medical illness.

Sometimes even it becomes difficult for a doctor to find reason behind increased anxiety. A psychologist and dance movement therapist must work together so that the level of anxiety in an individual can be controlled. It is important to control impulsivity, anger and other emotional imbalance related issues. The use of DMT can be used to control intense negative emotions, impulsivity, mood disorders and other related issues which are a potential cause for substance abuse, suicidal ideation, suicidal attempts and depression. It also hampers one's interpersonal relationships.

- **Obesity and Chronic Illnesses:** Obesity is a major cause for many other chronic illnesses. The present and many other researchers have concluded that dance is very beneficial for our psychophysical health. The use of dance as a form of physical exercise must be a part of various personality development programs. It is considered as a type of exercise. Nowadays, importance of Zumba which is type of dance has been increased for improving physical fitness. Apart from this importance of Aerobics dance form, Bollywood dance in physical fitness has been increased. Dance not only helps in reducing our body weight and physical fitness but it also helps us to be mentally fit. Dance as a form of exercise is useful in controlling obesity and other health and fitness related issues.

- **Physical Health Improvement:** Researches show that along with physical health it is very important to be mentally fit in one's life. It is should always be taken into consideration that how we think? How we feel? How we act in different situation which shows our mental health. With the help of dance, the mental health of peoples of different age groups; children, adults or senior citizens, their health and cognitive abilities can be improved. Dance enhances release of Dopamine and Endorphins in our body and these neurotransmitters are responsible for our pleasure feeling and happiness. Dance is not only beneficial for children and teenagers but is also beneficial for adults and old aged person. A study conducted on persons belonging to age group of 65-91 years in North Dakota reveals that dance improves mood and cognitive health of elderly persons as well. Dance therapy is recommended for the people who are suffering from obesity, depression, stress or anxiety. A dance class or exercise class or even in performing dance is also beneficial for healthy living.

- **Hospitals, Schools and Workplace Settings:** A counsellor in schools should organise dance sessions for the cognitive development, social skills and for overall personality development. Psychologist should organise dance session for the patients in hospitals who are suffering from any disease or illness and admitted in hospitals since a long time so their disease related anxiety can be reduced if it prevails in them. Dance sessions need to be open not only for person having physical illness but also for the healthy people who want to get benefitted by the dance and movement therapy. The companies should also organise dance sessions 1 or 2 times in a month for their employees with the help of psychologist who are trained in dance movement therapy. Also, the dance therapy should be given in old-age home, orphanage, deaf and dumb schools and NGOs etc so there mental and physical health can be improved.

- **Fostering Creativity & Innovation:** Dance is not only like performing high energy movements on high beats but it can also be soft and relaxing. We can say that dance is form of expression. From ancient times people of different communities and tribes expresses their thoughts and sentiments though dance. It is seen that dance enhances our creativity level. Dance and DMT can be used to foster creativity.

- **Fun Learning:** In academic settings also, dance can be incorporated as a fun way of learning. The use of dance along with the academic content can be used in creative way for children and specially-abled children so that their learning experiences can be improved and eased.

5.2 SUGGESTIONS

- The present research has studied the effect of dance on personality, anxiety and health. Some other variables can also be selected as dependent variables such as Creativity, Memory, Emotional Intelligence, Body Image, Interpersonal relationships, level of concentration, attention, cognitive functioning, Well-being etc.

- It is suggested that the future researchers focus on studies the difference in the effect of specific dance forms. Different groups can be provided specific dance forms and the comparison of these dance forms can also be planned.

- The sample consisted of the population in the age group of 18-30 years only. The further research must select sample from the other age groups i.e. children, middle age, elderly people so that the effect of dance on their health and other variables can also be understood.
- The present research has been conducted in the urban settings. Future research can be planned on the rural population also.
- Some specific studies are suggested for the dancers, choreographers who have been involved in dance since more than 5-10 years so that the effect of long term involvement in dance can also be understood. Comparative studies of dancers and non-dancers on various parameters would be more precisely understood when the sample of dancers has undergone long-term training/involvement in dance.
- There is a need to conduct researches which compare Indian and Western dance forms and its effect on the physical health, mental health, personality and other psychological variables. The research studying the effect of Kathak, Bharatnatyam, Kuchipudi and other classical dance forms on the various psychological parameters such as moods, emotional regulation, communication, level of confidence, self esteem, cognitive functioning etc can also be conducted.
- The Intervention Model used in this research has been implemented for four weeks. It is recommended that the future researchers could increase the duration of dance movement therapy intervention to gain a better output after the intervention.
- Some other population groups can also be provided dance movement therapy. The future researchers can conduct studies on the children, elderly population, juvenile delinquents, individuals/children who have suicidal ideations/attempts history and the patients of some specific diseases. The use of dance and other art forms as a way of obtaining deeper information need to be studied.

5.3 LIMITATIONS

- The present research has certain limitations related to the sample selected. The sample consisted of 120 adolescents only. The increase in the sample size would help in getting more generalized findings.
- There were some geographical constraints in the sample which is taken only from Udaipur while the sample from outside Udaipur can also be taken. For a more generalized findings, a research on the wider geographical area could be conducted.
- The sample taken was of the persons of the age group between 18-30 groups while the people from the others age group below or above this age group can also be studies to the effect of dance and dance movement therapy on various psychological variables. The findings of this research are applicable on the adolescents only.
- The intervention of dance movement therapy was also conducted on 20 adolescents; with 10 adolescents in each group i.e. control group and experimental group.

CPSIA information can be obtained
at www.ICGtesting.com
Printed in the USA
BVHW092017060822
643973BV00009B/932

9 781055 492163